MCAT®
POWER PRACTICE

MCAT®
POWER PRACTICE

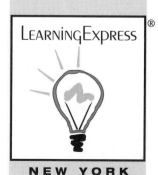

NEW YORK

For more information on LearningExpress, other LearningExpress products, or bulk sales,
please write to us at:
  80 Broad Street
  4th Floor
  New York, NY 10004

CONTENTS

1 ▶ ABOUT THE MCAT® EXAM

The Medical College Admission Test® (MCAT®) is designed to measure your ability to think critically and solve problems, and assess your knowledge base in a variety of core topic areas that are important to the study and field of medicine. If you're interested in attending medical school, you'll almost certainly have to take the MCAT® exam—and in this ultra-competitive environment you'll certainly want to get your best possible score.

The MCAT® exam has undergone a *major* overhaul in 2015, but don't worry—you've made a wise decision by getting this book! You'll get a complete overview of what the new MCAT® exam is like and everything you need to do between now and test day—from how to register to what to bring and everything in between—as well as test practice that's modeled on the official exam. Use *MCAT® Power Practice* as part of your MCAT® study plan, and you'll be well on your way to succeeding on test day and one step closer to achieving your goal of getting into medical school!

The MCAT® Exam:
What to Expect

The MCAT® exam is a multiple-choice test that's divided into four main test sections:

- Chemical and Physical Foundations of Biological Systems
- Psychological, Social, and Biological Foundations of Behavior
- Biological and Biochemical Foundations of Living Systems
- Critical Analysis and Reasoning Skills

We'll explore each test section in depth later in this chapter, so you'll know exactly what to expect and so you can prepare to get your best possible scores.

How the MCAT® Exam Is Scored

Your official MCAT® exam score will be a sum total of your scores on each of the four test sections. You will receive a score between 118 and 132 for each section, and your total score will range from 472 to 528. Good news—*there's no penalty for guessing*—so when you encounter challenging questions make sure you give them a shot, eliminating choices you know aren't correct in an effort to boost your chances of guessing correctly.

After completing the MCAT® exam, you can view your score report on the official Association of American Medical Colleges (AAMC) website (www.aamc.org) approximately one month after your test date.

- **AMCAS® participating institutions:** Your scores will be released automatically to the American College Application Service (AMCAS®), so if you're a prospective first-year student no additional action is required by you to include your scores as part of your online application to

medical school. If you're a prospective transfer student or advanced standing applicant, you should contact the schools to which you're applying for application guidelines.
- **Non-AMCAS® participating institutions:** Your MCAT® exam score can be sent to another application service or directly to a specific school, either electronically or via mail. Please visit the AAMC website for additional information.

Your score on the MCAT® exam is typically valid for 2–3 years, but this varies by institution. Please contact the medical school(s) you plan on applying to for their score acceptance policies.

Registering for the MCAT® Exam

If you're interested in earning a professional health degree, chances are you'll need to submit an MCAT® exam score as part of your school application.

In order to register for the MCAT® exam, you'll need to create an AAMC account and obtain an AAMC ID, username, and password. Visit the official AAMC website to create your account—and read and follow all of the directions *carefully*. This will also allow you to access additional MCAT®-related information and services.

Once you create your account, you'll be able to view a list of testing locations and schedules and register for an exam online through the AAMC's MCAT Scheduling and Registration System. The AAMC recommends that you register at least 60 days prior to your preferred test date.

For a complete list of registration and scheduling options and associated fees—including fee assistance—visit the official AAMC website (www.aamc.org). You'll also find helpful information on accommodated testing options if you have a disability or medical condition.

The MCAT® Exam—Test Overview

As previously mentioned, the MCAT® exam is a multiple-choice test that's divided into four main sections:

- Chemical and Physical Foundations of Biological Systems
- Psychological, Social, and Biological Foundations of Behavior
- Biological and Biochemical Foundations of Living Systems
- Critical Analysis and Reasoning Skills

The total exam time is 6 hours and 15 minutes, and the total "seated" time is 7 hours and 33 minutes—this includes the examinee agreement, optional tutorial, scheduled breaks between exam sections, and the void question and satisfaction survey at the end of the exam. (Please note that the exam includes a number of experimental items that don't count towards your score).

Let's look at each test section in a little more depth.

Chemical and Physical Foundations of Biological Systems

- Total number of questions: 59
  - 10 passage-based question sets (4–6 questions per set)
  - 15 independent questions (not passage based)
- Total time: 95 minutes

This section of the exam includes questions that assess your knowledge of core chemical and physical science concepts, along with your reasoning and scientific inquiry abilities. The questions you'll find in this section are based on college-level concepts in biology, biochemistry, general and organic chemistry, and physics.

Psychological, Social, and Biological Foundations of Behavior

- Total number of questions: 59
  - 10 passage-based question sets (4–6 questions per set)
  - 15 independent questions (not passage based)
- Total time: 95 minutes

This section of the exam includes questions that assess your knowledge of core psychological (consistent with DSM-5), social, and biological concepts, along with your reasoning and scientific inquiry abilities. The questions you'll find in this section are based on college-level concepts in biology, psychology, and sociology.

Biological and Biochemical Foundations of Living Systems

- Total number of questions: 59
  - 10 passage-based question sets (4–6 questions per set)
  - 15 independent questions (not passage based)
- Total time: 95 minutes

This section of the exam includes questions that assess your knowledge of core biological and biochemical concepts, along with your reasoning and scientific inquiry abilities. The questions you'll find in this section are based on college-level concepts in biology, biochemistry, and general and organic chemistry.

Critical Analysis and Reasoning Skills

- Total number of questions: 53
  - 9 passage-based question sets (5–7 questions per set)
- Total time: 90 minutes

This section of the exam includes questions that assess your ability to think critically, comprehend, assess, analyze, and reason through a variety of written material, which spans a wide array of academic disciplines across the humanities and social sciences.

Test Day Checklist

There's nothing worse than studying hard and preparing for an important exam like the MCAT®, only to have a small test day detail trip you up! Review the following list carefully and make sure you're prepared. Also be sure to visit the official AAMC website for all the information you need to know between now and test day.

❑ **Date and time:** Make sure you know the precise date and time of your exam. Write it down and make yourself a reminder. You certainly don't want to show up on the wrong day or after your exam has already begun!

❑ **Address:** Make sure you know the precise address of your test location and the most efficient route for getting there on time.

❑ **Transportation:** Are you getting to the test center by car? Bus? Train? Walking? Know your plan of attack for getting to your test center and make sure there are no unaccounted for variables (i.e., road construction causing traffic delays, etc.) that can derail your plans. Plan carefully and well ahead of time!

❑ **Arrival:** This is *important*—you must report to your test center at least 30 minutes prior to the start of your exam in order to be admitted. This extra time is used for the test center staff to verify your ID and seat assignment, and review and implement all required admissions procedures.

❑ **Bring your ID:** Just as important as being prepared to ace the MCAT® exam, make sure you bring acceptable ID on test day. This must be a current, government-issued ID that includes your signature and photo.

❑ **Dress comfortably:** Dress in comfortable layers so you can adjust to varying room temperature, and stay relaxed throughout the exam.

❑ **Listen:** On exam day, the test center staff will review all of the directions, rules, and procedures for taking the MCAT® exam. Make sure you listen *carefully* to everything you're told. Failure to follow the rules may have serious consequences.

❑ **The night before:** Make sure you get plenty of rest the night before the exam, and have a good, nutritious breakfast in the morning. Resist the urge to have an all-night, sugar-fueled cram session. This will not put you in your best test-taking shape!

❑ **What not to bring:** Leave the following at home on test day, or be prepared to have them stowed away in a secure location:
  ○ Food and beverages
  ○ A watch or timer
  ○ A cell phone or other electronic devices
  ○ Hats and scarves

Using this Book for MCAT® Exam Success

This book provides concentrated practice to get you ready for test day. We recommend that you use it as part of your overall MCAT® exam study plan, to determine your strengths and weaknesses in each test section and guide your further study and preparation.

Remember, practice and preparation are the keys to doing well on the MCAT® exam. Use this book to your advantage and make the most of your study time between now and test day. Good luck!

2 ▶ THE LEARNINGEXPRESS TEST PREPARATION SYSTEM

I t takes significant preparation to score well on any exam, and MCAT® is no exception. The LearningExpress Test Preparation System, developed by experts exclusively for LearningExpress, offers a number of strategies designed to facilitate the development of the skills, disciplines, and attitudes necessary for success.

Preparing for and attaining a passing score on the MCAT® exam requires surmounting an assortment of obstacles. While some may prove more troublesome than others, all of them carry the potential to hinder your performance and negatively affect your scores. Here are some examples:

- lack of familiarity with the exam format
- paralyzing test anxiety
- leaving preparation to the last minute
- not preparing at all

- failure to develop vital test-taking skills:
  - effectively pacing through an exam
  - using the process of elimination to answer questions accurately
  - knowing when and how to guess
- mental and/or physical fatigue
- test day blunders:
  - arriving late at the testing facility
  - taking the exam on an empty stomach
  - not accounting for fluctuations in temperature at the testing facility

The common thread among these obstacles is control. While a host of pressing, unanticipated, and sometimes unavoidable difficulties may frustrate your preparation, there remain some proven, effective strategies for placing yourself in the best possible position on exam day. These strategies can significantly improve your level of comfort with the exam, offering you not only the confidence you'll need, but also, and perhaps most importantly, a higher test score.

The LearningExpress Test Preparation System helps to put you in greater control. Separated into nine steps, the system heightens your confidence level by helping you understand both the exam and your own particular set of test-taking strengths and weaknesses. It helps you structure a study plan, practice a number of effective test-taking skills, and avoid mental and physical fatigue on exam day. Each step is accompanied by an activity.

While the following list suggests an approximate time for the completion of each step, these are only guidelines for your initial introduction. The regular practice of a number of them may require a more substantial time commitment. It may also be necessary and helpful to return to one or more of them throughout the course of your preparation.

Step 1.	Get information.	1 hour
Step 2.	Conquer test anxiety.	20 minutes
Step 3.	Make a plan.	20 minutes
Step 4.	Learn to manage your time.	10 minutes
Step 5.	Learn to use the process of elimination.	20 minutes
Step 6.	Reach your peak performance zone.	10 minutes
Step 7.	Make final preparations.	10 minutes
Step 8.	Make your preparations count.	10 minutes
Total		2 hours, 40 minutes

We estimate that working through the entire system will take you approximately three hours. It's perfectly okay if you work at a faster or slower pace. It's up to you to decide whether you should set aside a whole afternoon or evening to work through the LearningExpress Test Preparation System in one sitting, or break it up and do just one or two steps a day for the next several days.

Step 1: Get Information

Time to complete: 1 hour
Activities: Read the introduction to this book.

Knowing more about an exam can often make it appear less daunting. The first step in the Learning Express Test Preparation System is to determine everything you can about the type of information you will be expected to know on the MCAT® exam, as well as how your knowledge will be assessed.

What You Should Find Out

Knowing the details will help you study efficiently and help you feel a sense of control. Here's a list of things you might want to find out:

- What skills are tested?
- How many sections are on the exam?
- How many questions are in each section?
- How much time is allotted for each section?
- How is the exam scored, and is there a penalty for guessing/wrong answers?
- Is the test computerized or will you have an exam booklet?
- Will you be given scratch paper to write on?

You will find answers to these questions in Chapter 1 of this book and on the NCSBN's MCAT® website, www.ncsbn.org.

Step 2: Conquer Test Anxiety

Time to complete: 20 minutes
Activity: Take the Test Stress Quiz.

Now that you know what's on the test, the next step is to address one of the biggest obstacles to success: *test anxiety*. Test anxiety may not only impair your performance on the exam itself, but it can also keep you from preparing properly. In Step 2, you will learn stress management techniques that will help you succeed on your exam. Practicing these techniques as you work through the activities in this book will help them become second nature to you by exam day.

Combating Test Anxiety

A little test anxiety is a good thing. Everyone gets nervous before a big exam—and if that nervousness motivates you to prepare thoroughly, so much the better. Many athletes report pregame jitters, which they are able to harness to help them perform at their peak. Stop here and answer the questions on the Test Stress Quiz that follows to determine your level of test anxiety.

Stress Management before the Exam

If you feel your level of anxiety is getting the best of you in the weeks before the exam, here are things you can do to bring the level down:

- **Prepare.** There's nothing like knowing what to expect to put you in control of test anxiety. That's why you're reading this book. Use it faithfully, and you will be ready on test day.
- **Practice self-confidence.** A positive attitude is a great way to combat test anxiety. Stand in front of the mirror and say to your reflection, "I'm prepared. I'm confident. I'm going to ace this exam. I know I can do it." As soon as negative thoughts creep in, drown them out with these positive affirmations. If you hear them often enough, and you use the LearningExpress method to study for MCAT®, they will be true.
- **Fight negative messages.** Every time someone talks to you about how hard the exam is or says it's difficult to pass, think about your self-confidence messages. If the someone with the negative messages is you—you're telling yourself you don't do well on exams, that you just can't do this—don't listen. Repeat self-confidence messages.
- **Visualize.** Visualizing success can help make it happen, and it reminds you of why you're doing all this work in preparing for the exam. Imagine yourself in your first day of classes or beginning the first day of your dream job.
- **Exercise.** Physical activity helps calm your body and focus your mind. Besides, being in good physical shape can actually help you do well on the exam. Go for a run, lift weights, go swimming—and exercise regularly.

You need to worry about test anxiety only if it is extreme enough to impair your performance. The following questionnaire provides a diagnosis of your level of test anxiety. In the blank before each statement, write the number that most accurately describes your experience.

0 = Never
1 = Once or twice
2 = Sometimes
3 = Often

___ I have gotten so nervous before an exam that I simply put down the books and didn't study for it.

___ I have experienced disabling physical symptoms such as vomiting and severe headaches because I was nervous about an exam.

___ I have simply not showed up for an exam because I was scared to take it.

___ I have experienced dizziness and disorientation while taking an exam.

___ I have had trouble filling in the little circles because my hands were shaking too hard.

___ I have failed an exam because I was too nervous to complete it.

___ **Total: Add up the numbers in the blanks.**

Your Test Stress Score

Here are the steps you should take, depending on your score. If you scored:

- **Below 3,** your level of test anxiety is nothing to worry about; it's probably just enough to give you that extra edge.

- **Between 3 and 6,** your test anxiety may be enough to impair your performance, and you should practice the stress-management techniques in this section to try to bring your test anxiety down to manageable levels.

- **Above 6,** your level of test anxiety is a serious concern. In addition to practicing the stress management techniques listed in this section, you may want to seek additional, personal help. Call your community college and ask for the academic counselor or ask the counselor at your nursing school. Tell the counselor that you have a level of test anxiety that sometimes keeps you from being able to take the exam. The counselor may be willing to help you or may suggest someone else you should talk to.

Stress Management on Test Day

There are several ways you can bring down your level of test stress and anxiety on test day. They'll work best if you practice them in the weeks before the exam, so you know which ones work best for you.

- **Breathe deeply.** Take a deep breath in while you count to five. Hold it for a count of one, and then let it out on a count of five. Repeat several times.
- **Move your body.** Try rolling your head in a circle. Rotate your shoulders. Shake your hands from the wrist.
- **Visualize again.** Think of the place where you are most relaxed: lying on the beach in the sun, walking through the park, or wherever relaxes you. Now, close your eyes and imagine you're actually there. If you practice in advance, you will find that you need only a few seconds of this exercise to experience a significant increase in your sense of relaxation and well-being.

When anxiety threatens to overwhelm you during the test, there are still things you can do to manage your stress level:

- **Repeat your self-confidence messages.** You should have them memorized by now. Say them quietly to yourself, and believe them!
- **Visualize one more time.** This time, visualize yourself moving smoothly and quickly through the exam, answering every question correctly, and finishing just before time is up. Like most visualization techniques, this one works best if you've practiced it ahead of time.
- **Find an easy question.** Skim over the questions until you find an easy one, and then answer it. Getting even one question answered correctly gets you into the test-taking groove.

- **Take a mental break.** Everyone loses concentration once in a while during a long exam. It's normal, so you shouldn't worry about it. Instead, accept what has happened. Say to yourself, "Hey, I lost it there for a minute. My brain is taking a break." Close your eyes and do some deep breathing for a few seconds. Then go back to work.

Try these techniques ahead of time and see whether they work for you!

Step 3: Make a Plan

Time to complete: 20 minutes
Activity: Construct a study plan.

There is no substitute for careful preparation and practice over time. So the most important thing you can do to better prepare yourself for your exam is to create a study plan or schedule and then follow it. This will help you avoid cramming at the last minute, which is an ineffective study technique that will only add to your anxiety.

Once you make your plan, make a commitment to follow it. Set aside at least 30 minutes every day for studying and practice. This will do more good than two hours crammed into a Saturday. If you have months before the test, you're lucky. Don't put off your studying until the week before. Start now. Even 10 minutes on weekdays, with half an hour or more on weekends, can make a big difference in your score.

Step 4: Learn to Manage Your Time

Time to complete: 10 minutes to read, many hours of practice
Activities: Practice these strategies as you take the sample exams.

Steps 4, 5, and 6 of the LearningExpress Test Preparation System put you in charge of your MCAT® experience by showing you test-taking strategies that work. Practice these strategies as you take the practice exams in this book and online. Then, you will be ready to use them on test day.

First, you will take control of your time on MCAT®. Start by understanding the format of the test. Refer to Chapter 1 to review this information; in particular, make sure you understand the way the computerized adaptive testing (CAT) works.

You will want to practice using your time wisely on the practice tests, while trying to avoid making mistakes while working quickly.

- **Listen carefully to directions.** By the time you get to the test, you should know how it works. But listen carefully in case something has changed.
- **Pace yourself.** Glance at your watch every few minutes to ensure that you are not taking much more than one to two minutes on each question.
- **Keep moving.** Don't spend too much time on one question. If you don't know the answer, skip the question and move on. Mark the question for review and come back to it later, if possible.
- **Don't rush.** You should keep moving, but rushing won't help. Try to keep calm and work methodically and quickly.

Step 5: Learn to Use the Process of Elimination

Time to complete: 20 minutes
Activity: Complete worksheet on the process of elimination.

After time management, the next most important tool for taking control of your test is using the process of elimination wisely. It's standard test-taking wisdom that you should always read all the answer choices before choosing your answer. This helps you find the right answer by eliminating wrong answer choices. Consider the following question. Although it is not the type of question you will see on MCAT®, the mental process that you use will be the same.

> **Sentence 6:** I would like to be considered for the assistant manager position in your company my previous work experience is a good match for the job requirements posted.
> Which correction should be made to sentence 6?
> **a.** Insert *Although* before *I*.
> **b.** Insert a question mark after *company*.
> **c.** Insert a semicolon and *however* before *my*.
> **d.** Insert a period after *company* and capitalize *my*.
> **e.** No corrections are necessary.

If you happen to know that sentence 6 is a run-on sentence, and you know how to correct it, you don't need to use the process of elimination. But let's assume that, like some people, you don't. So, you look at the answer choices. *Although* sure doesn't sound like a good choice, because it would change the meaning of the sentence. So, you eliminate choice **a**, and now you only have four answer choices to deal with.

Write **a** on your note board with an X through or beside it. Move on to the other answer choices.

If you know that the first part of the sentence does not ask a question, you can eliminate choice **b** as a possible answer. Write **b** on your note board with an X through or beside it. Choice **c**, inserting a semicolon, could create a pause in an otherwise long sentence, but inserting the word *however* might not be correct. If you're not sure whether this answer is correct, write **c** on your note board with a question mark beside it, meaning "well, maybe."

Choice **d** would separate a very long sentence into two shorter sentences, and it would not change the meaning. It could work, so write **d** on your note board with a check mark beside it, meaning "good answer." Choice **e** means that the sentence is fine like it is and doesn't need any changes. The sentence could make sense as it is, but it is definitely long. Is this the best way to write the sentence? If you're not sure, write **e** on your note board with a question mark beside it.

Now, your note board looks like this:

X **a.**
X **b.**
? **c.**
✓ **d.**
? **e.**

You've got just one check mark, for a good answer, **d**. If you're pressed for time, you should simply select choice **d**. If you've got the time to be extra careful, you could compare your check mark answer to your question mark answers to make sure that it's better. (It is: Sentence 6 is a run-on, and should be separated into two shorter, complete sentences.)

It's good to have a system for marking good, bad, and maybe answers. We recommend using this one:

X = bad
✓ = good
? = maybe

If you don't like these marks, devise your own system. Just make sure you do it long before exam day—while you're working through the practice tests in this book and online—so you won't have to worry about it during the exam.

Even when you think you're absolutely clueless about a question, you can use the process of elimination to get rid of one answer choice. By doing so, you're better prepared to make an educated guess. Often, the process of elimination allows you to get down to only two possible right answers. Nevertheless, as explained in Chapter 1, rapid guessing is a strategy that should be avoided in the MCAT®. It will result in the computer program giving candidates easier items, which you may also get wrong if you are guessing and running short on time.

Try using your powers of elimination on the following questions. The answer explanations show one possible way you might use the process to arrive at the right answer.

Step 6: Reach Your Peak Performance Zone

Time to complete: 10 minutes to read, weeks to complete!
Activity: Complete the Physical Preparation Checklist.

Physical and mental fatigue can significantly hinder your ability to perform not only as you prepare, but also on the day of the exam. Poor diet choices can hinder you, as well. Drastic changes to your existing daily routine may cause a disruption too great to be helpful, but modest, calculated alterations in your level of physical activity, the quality of your diet, and the amount and regularity of your rest can enhance your studies and your performance on the exam.

USING THE PROCESS OF ELIMINATION

Use the process of elimination to answer the following questions.

1. Ilsa is as old as Meghan will be in five years. The difference between Ed's age and Meghan's age is twice the difference between Ilsa's age and Meghan's age. Ed is 29. How old is Ilsa?
   a. 4
   b. 10
   c. 19
   d. 24

2. "All drivers of commercial vehicles must carry a valid commercial driver's license whenever operating a commercial vehicle."
   According to this sentence, which of the following people need NOT carry a commercial driver's license?
   a. a truck driver idling his engine while waiting to be directed to a loading dock
   b. a bus operator backing her bus out of the way of another bus in the bus lot
   c. a taxi driver driving his personal car to the grocery store
   d. a limousine driver taking the limousine to her home after dropping off her last passenger of the evening

3. Smoking tobacco has been linked to
   a. increased risk of stroke and heart attack.
   b. all forms of respiratory disease.
   c. increasing mortality rates over the past 10 years.
   d. juvenile delinquency.

4. Which of the following words is spelled correctly?
   a. incorrigible
   b. outragous
   c. domestickated
   d. understandible

Answers

Here are the answers, as well as some suggestions as to how you might have used the process of elimination to find them.

1. d. You should have eliminated choice **a** right off the bat. Ilsa can't be four years old if Meghan is going to be Ilsa's age in five years. The best way to eliminate other answer choices is to try plugging them into the information given in the problem. For instance, for choice **b**, if Ilsa is 10, then Meghan must be 5. The difference between their ages is 5. The difference between Ed's age, 29, and Meghan's age, 5, is 24. Is 24 two times 5? No. Then choice **b** is wrong. You could eliminate choice **c** in the same way and be left with choice **d**.

2. c. Note the word not in the question, and go through the answers one by one. Is the truck driver in choice **a** "operating a commercial vehicle"? Yes, idling counts as "operating," so he needs to have a commercial driver's license. Likewise, the bus operator in choice **b** is operating a commercial vehicle; the question doesn't say the operator has to be on the street. The limo driver in choice **d** is operating a commercial vehicle, even if it doesn't have a passenger in it. However, the driver in choice **c** is not operating a commercial vehicle, but his own private car.

3. a. You could eliminate choice **b** simply because of the presence of the word *all*. Such absolutes hardly ever appear in correct answer choices. Choice **c** looks attractive until you think a little about what you know—aren't fewer people smoking these days, rather than more? So how could smoking be responsible for a higher mortality rate? (If you didn't know that mortality rate means the rate at which people die, you might keep this choice as a possibility, but you would still be able to eliminate two answers and have only two to choose from.) And choice **d** is plain silly, so you could eliminate that one, too. You are left with the correct choice, **a**.

4. a. How you used the process of elimination here depends on which words you recognized as being spelled incorrectly. If you knew that the correct spellings were *outrageous*, *domesticated*, and *understandable*, then you would be home free. Surely you knew that at least one of those words was wrong in the question!

Exercise

If you are already engaged in a regular program of physical activity, resist allowing the pressure of the approaching exam to alter this routine. If you are not, and have not been engaged in regular physical activity, it may be helpful to begin during your preparations. Speak with someone knowledgeable about such matters to design a regimen suited to your particular circumstances and needs. Whatever its form, try to keep it a regular part of your preparation as the exam approaches.

Diet

A balanced diet will help you achieve peak performance. Limit your caffeine and junk food intake as you continue on your preparation journey. Eat plenty

The following are ten really hard questions. You are not supposed to know the answers. Rather, this is an assessment of your ability to guess when you don't have a clue. Read each question carefully, as if you were expected to answer it. If you have any knowledge of the subject, use that knowledge to help you eliminate wrong answer choices.

1. September 7 is Independence Day in
   a. India.
   b. Costa Rica.
   c. Brazil.
   d. Australia.

2. Which of the following is the formula for determining the momentum of an object?
   a. $p = MV$
   b. $F = ma$
   c. $P = IV$
   d. $E = mc^2$

3. Because of the expansion of the universe, the stars and other celestial bodies are all moving away from each other. This phenomenon is known as
   a. Newton's first law.
   b. the big bang.
   c. gravitational collapse.
   d. Hubble flow.

4. American author Gertrude Stein was born in
   a. 1713.
   b. 1830.
   c. 1874.
   d. 1901.

5. Which of the following is NOT one of the Five Classics attributed to Confucius?
   a. *I Ching*
   b. *Book of Holiness*
   c. *Spring and Autumn Annals*
   d. *Book of History*

6. The religious and philosophical doctrine that holds that the universe is constantly in a struggle between good and evil is known as
   a. Pelagianism.
   b. Manichaeanism.
   c. neo-Hegelianism.
   d. Epicureanism.

7. The third Chief Justice of the U.S. Supreme Court was
   a. John Blair.
   b. William Cushing.
   c. James Wilson.
   d. John Jay.

8. Which of the following is the poisonous portion of a daffodil?
   a. the bulb
   b. the leaves
   c. the stem
   d. the flowers

9. The winner of the Masters golf tournament in 1953 was
   a. Sam Snead.
   b. Cary Middlecoff.
   c. Arnold Palmer.
   d. Ben Hogan.

10. The state with the highest per capita personal income in 1980 was
    a. Alaska.
    b. Connecticut.
    c. New York.
    d. Texas.

Answers

Check your answers against the following correct answers.

1. c.
2. a.
3. d.
4. c.
5. b.
6. b.
7. b.
8. a.
9. d.
10. a.

How Did You Do?

You may have simply gotten lucky and actually known the answer to one or two questions. In addition, your guessing was probably more successful if you were able to use the process of elimination on any of the questions. Maybe you didn't know who the third Chief Justice was (question 7), but you knew that John Jay was the first. In that case, you would have eliminated choice **d** and, therefore, improved your odds of guessing right from one in four to one in three.

According to probability, you should get two-and-a-half answers correct, so getting either two or three right would be average. If you got four or more right, you may be a really terrific guesser. If you got one or none right, you may be a really bad guesser.

Keep in mind, though, that this is only a small sample. You should continue to keep track of your guessing ability as you work through the sample questions in this book. Circle the numbers of questions you guess on as you make your guess; or, if you don't have time while you take the practice tests, go back afterward and try to remember which questions you guessed at. Remember, on a test with four answer choices, your chance of guessing correctly is one in four. So keep a separate "guessing" score for each exam. How many questions did you guess on? How many did you get right? If the number you got right is at least one-fourth of the number of questions you guessed on, you are at least an average guesser—maybe better—and you should always go ahead and guess on the real exam. If the number you got right is significantly lower than one-fourth of the number you guessed on, you would be safe in guessing anyway, but maybe you would feel more comfortable if you guessed only selectively, when you can eliminate a wrong answer or at least have a good feeling about one of the answer choices.

Remember, even if you are a play-it-safe person with lousy intuition, you are still safe guessing every time.

of fruits and vegetables, along with lean proteins and complex carbohydrates. Foods that are high in lecithin (an amino acid), such as fish and beans, are especially good brain foods.

Your diet is also a matter that is particular to you, so any major alterations to it should be discussed with a person with expert knowledge of nutrition.

Rest

For your brain and body to function at optimal levels, they must have an adequate amount of rest. It is important to determine what an adequate amount of rest is for you. Determine how much rest you need to feel at your sharpest and most alert, and make an effort to get that amount regularly as the exam approaches and particularly on the night before the exam.

It may help to record your efforts. What follows is a Physical Preparation Checklist for the week prior to the exam; you may find its use helpful for staying on track.

For the week before the test, record the type and duration of your physical exercise, your food consumption for each day, and the number of hours you slept.

Exam minus 7 days

Exercise: _____ for _____ minutes

Breakfast: _____

Lunch: _____

Dinner: _____

Snacks: _____

Sleep: _____

Exam minus 6 days

Exercise: _____ for _____ minutes

Breakfast: _____

Lunch: _____

Dinner: _____

Snacks: _____

Sleep: _____

Exam minus 5 days

Exercise: _____ for _____ minutes

Breakfast: _____

Lunch: _____

Dinner: _____

Snacks: _____

Sleep: _____

Exam minus 4 days

Exercise: _____ for _____ minutes

Breakfast: _____

Lunch: _____

Dinner: _____

Snacks: _____

Sleep: _____

Exam minus 3 days

Exercise: _____ for _____ minutes

Breakfast: _____

Lunch: _____

Dinner: _____

Snacks: _____

Sleep: _____

Exam minus 2 days

Exercise: _____ for _____ minutes

Breakfast: _____

Lunch: _____

Dinner: _____

Snacks: _____

Sleep: _____

Exam minus 1 day

Exercise: _____ for _____ minutes

Breakfast: _____

Lunch: _____

Dinner: _____

Snacks: _____

Sleep: _____

Physical Preparation Checklist

In the week leading up to the test, you may be so involved with studying (and, unfortunately, stress) that you neglect to treat your body kindly. The worksheet on the previous page will help you stay on track.

For each day of the week before the test, write down what physical exercise you engaged in and for how long, and what you ate for each meal. Remember, you're trying for at least half an hour of exercise every other day (preferably every day) and a balanced diet that is light on junk food. These practices are key to your body and brain working at their peak.

Step 7: Make Final Preparations

Time to complete: 10 minutes to read; time to complete will vary
Activity: Complete the Final Preparations worksheet.

You're in control of your mind and body; you're in charge of test anxiety, your preparation, and your test-taking strategies. Now, it's time to take charge of external factors, like the testing site and the materials you need to take the test.

Find Out Where the Exam Is and Make a Trial Run

Make sure you know exactly when and where your test is being held. Do you know how to get to the exam site? Do you know how long it will take to get there? If not, make a trial run if possible, preferably on the same day of the week at the same time of day. On the Final Preparations worksheet, make note of the amount of time it will take you to get to the test site. Plan on arriving at least 30 to 45 minutes early so you can get the lay of the land, use the bathroom, and calm down. Then figure out how early you will have to get up that morning, and make sure you get up that early every day for a week before the test.

Gather Your Materials

Make sure you have all the materials that will be required at the testing facility. Whether it's an admission ticket, two forms of ID, pencils, pens, calculators, a watch, or any other item that may be necessary, make sure you have put it aside. It's preferable to put them all aside together.

Arrange your clothes the evening before the exam. Dress in layers so that you can adjust readily to the temperature of the exam room.

Fuel Appropriately

Decide on a meal to eat in the time before your exam. Taking the exam on an empty stomach is something to avoid, particularly if it is an exam that spans several hours. Eating poorly and feeling lethargic are also to be avoided. Decide on a meal that will sate your hunger without adverse effect.

Final Preparations

To help get organized, a Final Preparations worksheet is included on page 19.

Step 8: Make Your Preparations Count

Time to complete: 10 minutes, plus test-taking time
Activity: Ace the MCAT®!

Fast-forward to test day. You're ready. You made a study plan and followed through. You practiced your test-taking strategies while working through this book. You're in control of your physical, mental, and emotional state. You know when and where to show up and what to bring with you. In other words, you're well prepared!

When you're finished with the test, you will have earned a reward. Plan a celebration. Call up your friends and plan a party, have a nice dinner with your family, or pick out a movie to see—whatever your heart desires.

And then do it. Go into the test full of confidence, armed with test-taking strategies you've practiced until they're second nature. You're in control of yourself, your environment, and your performance on the exam. You're ready to succeed. So do it. And look forward to your future as someone who has passed the MCAT®!

Getting to the exam site:

Exam date: _____

Location of exam site: _____

Do I know how to get to the exam site?   Yes ___   No ___   (If no, make a trial run.)

Time it will take to get to the exam site: _____

Departure time: _____

Things to Lay Out the Night Before

Clothes I will wear   ____

Sweater/jacket   ____

Photo ID   ____

Four #2 pencils   ____

Other Things to Bring/Remember

_____   _____

_____   _____

_____   _____

_____   _____

3 ▶ MCAT® EXAM PRACTICE TEST 1

CHAPTER SUMMARY
This is the first of two practice MCAT® exams.

The exam is organized in four parts:

- Part 1: Biological and Biochemical Foundations of Living Systems
- Part 2: Chemical and Physical Foundations of Biological Systems
- Part 3: Psychological, Social, and Biological Foundations of Behavior
- Part 4: Critical Analysis and Reasoning Skills

(Note: you will have access to the Periodic Table of Elements during the exam.)

This practice test is modeled on the content, format, and length of the official MCAT® exam. At the beginning of each section you'll find the number of questions and time allotted. We recommend that you take the test under timed conditions, so you can get an accurate assessment of how you might do on test day, and determine the pace you'll need to work at.

Use your results on each section of the exam to determine your strengths and weaknesses, and guide your study. Good luck!

Part 1: Biological and Biochemical Foundations of Living Systems

1.	ⓐ	ⓑ	ⓒ	ⓓ
2.	ⓐ	ⓑ	ⓒ	ⓓ
3.	ⓐ	ⓑ	ⓒ	ⓓ
4.	ⓐ	ⓑ	ⓒ	ⓓ
5.	ⓐ	ⓑ	ⓒ	ⓓ
6.	ⓐ	ⓑ	ⓒ	ⓓ
7.	ⓐ	ⓑ	ⓒ	ⓓ
8.	ⓐ	ⓑ	ⓒ	ⓓ
9.	ⓐ	ⓑ	ⓒ	ⓓ
10.	ⓐ	ⓑ	ⓒ	ⓓ
11.	ⓐ	ⓑ	ⓒ	ⓓ
12.	ⓐ	ⓑ	ⓒ	ⓓ
13.	ⓐ	ⓑ	ⓒ	ⓓ
14.	ⓐ	ⓑ	ⓒ	ⓓ
15.	ⓐ	ⓑ	ⓒ	ⓓ
16.	ⓐ	ⓑ	ⓒ	ⓓ
17.	ⓐ	ⓑ	ⓒ	ⓓ
18.	ⓐ	ⓑ	ⓒ	ⓓ
19.	ⓐ	ⓑ	ⓒ	ⓓ
20.	ⓐ	ⓑ	ⓒ	ⓓ
21.	ⓐ	ⓑ	ⓒ	ⓓ
22.	ⓐ	ⓑ	ⓒ	ⓓ
23.	ⓐ	ⓑ	ⓒ	ⓓ
24.	ⓐ	ⓑ	ⓒ	ⓓ
25.	ⓐ	ⓑ	ⓒ	ⓓ
26.	ⓐ	ⓑ	ⓒ	ⓓ
27.	ⓐ	ⓑ	ⓒ	ⓓ
28.	ⓐ	ⓑ	ⓒ	ⓓ
29.	ⓐ	ⓑ	ⓒ	ⓓ
30.	ⓐ	ⓑ	ⓒ	ⓓ
31.	ⓐ	ⓑ	ⓒ	ⓓ
32.	ⓐ	ⓑ	ⓒ	ⓓ
33.	ⓐ	ⓑ	ⓒ	ⓓ
34.	ⓐ	ⓑ	ⓒ	ⓓ
35.	ⓐ	ⓑ	ⓒ	ⓓ
36.	ⓐ	ⓑ	ⓒ	ⓓ
37.	ⓐ	ⓑ	ⓒ	ⓓ
38.	ⓐ	ⓑ	ⓒ	ⓓ
39.	ⓐ	ⓑ	ⓒ	ⓓ
40.	ⓐ	ⓑ	ⓒ	ⓓ
41.	ⓐ	ⓑ	ⓒ	ⓓ
42.	ⓐ	ⓑ	ⓒ	ⓓ
43.	ⓐ	ⓑ	ⓒ	ⓓ
44.	ⓐ	ⓑ	ⓒ	ⓓ
45.	ⓐ	ⓑ	ⓒ	ⓓ
46.	ⓐ	ⓑ	ⓒ	ⓓ
47.	ⓐ	ⓑ	ⓒ	ⓓ
48.	ⓐ	ⓑ	ⓒ	ⓓ
49.	ⓐ	ⓑ	ⓒ	ⓓ
50.	ⓐ	ⓑ	ⓒ	ⓓ
51.	ⓐ	ⓑ	ⓒ	ⓓ
52.	ⓐ	ⓑ	ⓒ	ⓓ
53.	ⓐ	ⓑ	ⓒ	ⓓ
54.	ⓐ	ⓑ	ⓒ	ⓓ
55.	ⓐ	ⓑ	ⓒ	ⓓ
56.	ⓐ	ⓑ	ⓒ	ⓓ
57.	ⓐ	ⓑ	ⓒ	ⓓ
58.	ⓐ	ⓑ	ⓒ	ⓓ
59.	ⓐ	ⓑ	ⓒ	ⓓ

Part 2: Chemical and Physical Foundations of Biological Systems

1.	ⓐ	ⓑ	ⓒ	ⓓ
2.	ⓐ	ⓑ	ⓒ	ⓓ
3.	ⓐ	ⓑ	ⓒ	ⓓ
4.	ⓐ	ⓑ	ⓒ	ⓓ
5.	ⓐ	ⓑ	ⓒ	ⓓ
6.	ⓐ	ⓑ	ⓒ	ⓓ
7.	ⓐ	ⓑ	ⓒ	ⓓ
8.	ⓐ	ⓑ	ⓒ	ⓓ
9.	ⓐ	ⓑ	ⓒ	ⓓ
10.	ⓐ	ⓑ	ⓒ	ⓓ
11.	ⓐ	ⓑ	ⓒ	ⓓ
12.	ⓐ	ⓑ	ⓒ	ⓓ
13.	ⓐ	ⓑ	ⓒ	ⓓ
14.	ⓐ	ⓑ	ⓒ	ⓓ
15.	ⓐ	ⓑ	ⓒ	ⓓ
16.	ⓐ	ⓑ	ⓒ	ⓓ
17.	ⓐ	ⓑ	ⓒ	ⓓ
18.	ⓐ	ⓑ	ⓒ	ⓓ
19.	ⓐ	ⓑ	ⓒ	ⓓ
20.	ⓐ	ⓑ	ⓒ	ⓓ
21.	ⓐ	ⓑ	ⓒ	ⓓ
22.	ⓐ	ⓑ	ⓒ	ⓓ
23.	ⓐ	ⓑ	ⓒ	ⓓ
24.	ⓐ	ⓑ	ⓒ	ⓓ
25.	ⓐ	ⓑ	ⓒ	ⓓ
26.	ⓐ	ⓑ	ⓒ	ⓓ
27.	ⓐ	ⓑ	ⓒ	ⓓ
28.	ⓐ	ⓑ	ⓒ	ⓓ
29.	ⓐ	ⓑ	ⓒ	ⓓ
30.	ⓐ	ⓑ	ⓒ	ⓓ
31.	ⓐ	ⓑ	ⓒ	ⓓ
32.	ⓐ	ⓑ	ⓒ	ⓓ
33.	ⓐ	ⓑ	ⓒ	ⓓ
34.	ⓐ	ⓑ	ⓒ	ⓓ
35.	ⓐ	ⓑ	ⓒ	ⓓ
36.	ⓐ	ⓑ	ⓒ	ⓓ
37.	ⓐ	ⓑ	ⓒ	ⓓ
38.	ⓐ	ⓑ	ⓒ	ⓓ
39.	ⓐ	ⓑ	ⓒ	ⓓ
40.	ⓐ	ⓑ	ⓒ	ⓓ
41.	ⓐ	ⓑ	ⓒ	ⓓ
42.	ⓐ	ⓑ	ⓒ	ⓓ
43.	ⓐ	ⓑ	ⓒ	ⓓ
44.	ⓐ	ⓑ	ⓒ	ⓓ
45.	ⓐ	ⓑ	ⓒ	ⓓ
46.	ⓐ	ⓑ	ⓒ	ⓓ
47.	ⓐ	ⓑ	ⓒ	ⓓ
48.	ⓐ	ⓑ	ⓒ	ⓓ
49.	ⓐ	ⓑ	ⓒ	ⓓ
50.	ⓐ	ⓑ	ⓒ	ⓓ
51.	ⓐ	ⓑ	ⓒ	ⓓ
52.	ⓐ	ⓑ	ⓒ	ⓓ
53.	ⓐ	ⓑ	ⓒ	ⓓ
54.	ⓐ	ⓑ	ⓒ	ⓓ
55.	ⓐ	ⓑ	ⓒ	ⓓ
56.	ⓐ	ⓑ	ⓒ	ⓓ
57.	ⓐ	ⓑ	ⓒ	ⓓ
58.	ⓐ	ⓑ	ⓒ	ⓓ
59.	ⓐ	ⓑ	ⓒ	ⓓ

Part 3: Psychological, Social, and Biological Foundations of Behavior

1.	a b c d		21.	a b c d		41.	a b c d
2.	a b c d		22.	a b c d		42.	a b c d
3.	a b c d		23.	a b c d		43.	a b c d
4.	a b c d		24.	a b c d		44.	a b c d
5.	a b c d		25.	a b c d		45.	a b c d
6.	a b c d		26.	a b c d		46.	a b c d
7.	a b c d		27.	a b c d		47.	a b c d
8.	a b c d		28.	a b c d		48.	a b c d
9.	a b c d		29.	a b c d		49.	a b c d
10.	a b c d		30.	a b c d		50.	a b c d
11.	a b c d		31.	a b c d		51.	a b c d
12.	a b c d		32.	a b c d		52.	a b c d
13.	a b c d		33.	a b c d		53.	a b c d
14.	a b c d		34.	a b c d		54.	a b c d
15.	a b c d		35.	a b c d		55.	a b c d
16.	a b c d		36.	a b c d		56.	a b c d
17.	a b c d		37.	a b c d		57.	a b c d
18.	a b c d		38.	a b c d		58.	a b c d
19.	a b c d		39.	a b c d		59.	a b c d
20.	a b c d		40.	a b c d			

Part 4: Critical Analysis and Reasoning Skills

1.	a b c d		19.	a b c d		37.	a b c d
2.	a b c d		20.	a b c d		38.	a b c d
3.	a b c d		21.	a b c d		39.	a b c d
4.	a b c d		22.	a b c d		40.	a b c d
5.	a b c d		23.	a b c d		41.	a b c d
6.	a b c d		24.	a b c d		42.	a b c d
7.	a b c d		25.	a b c d		43.	a b c d
8.	a b c d		26.	a b c d		44.	a b c d
9.	a b c d		27.	a b c d		45.	a b c d
10.	a b c d		28.	a b c d		46.	a b c d
11.	a b c d		29.	a b c d		47.	a b c d
12.	a b c d		30.	a b c d		48.	a b c d
13.	a b c d		31.	a b c d		49.	a b c d
14.	a b c d		32.	a b c d		50.	a b c d
15.	a b c d		33.	a b c d		51.	a b c d
16.	a b c d		34.	a b c d		52.	a b c d
17.	a b c d		35.	a b c d		53.	a b c d
18.	a b c d		36.	a b c d			

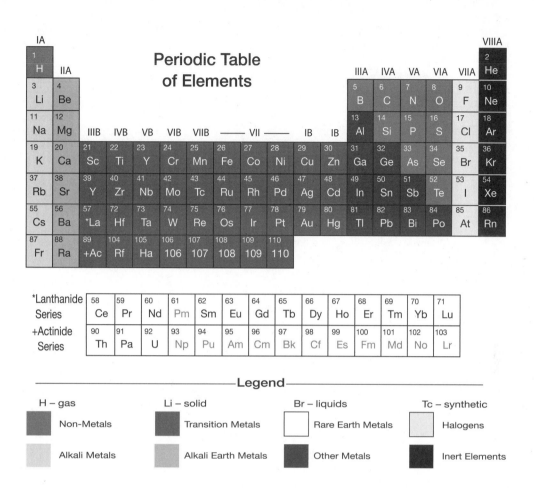

Periodic Table of Elements

Legend

H – gas
Non-Metals

Li – solid
Transition Metals

Br – liquids
Rare Earth Metals

Tc – synthetic
Halogens

Alkali Metals

Alkali Earth Metals

Other Metals

Inert Elements

Part 1: Biological and Biochemical Foundations of Living Systems

59 Questions
95 Minutes

Use the following passage to answer questions 1 through 4.

Hospitals and clinics in the United States and around the world face constant shortages in the supply of blood for transfusions. One alternative currently being explored is to make recombinant human hemoglobin (rHb). In addition to increasing supply for transfusions, rHb has a longer shelf life than red blood cells, is compatible with all blood types, and poses lower risk of transmitting disease. Despite these advantages, neither rHb products nor hemoglobin purified from animals has been licensed as therapy in the United States, mainly because of reports of hypertension and associated cardiovascular and cerebrovascular problems. (A product called HBOC-201, which is purified from cows, has been approved for human use in South Africa and Russia.) The toxicity of rHb has been attributed to the protein's presence in the plasma, where it can scavenge nitric oxide (NO), undergo oxidative reactions that damage tissues, denature,

aggregate, and precipitate, among other activities. In contrast, endogenous hemoglobin localizes in erythrocytes, where the cell membrane and cellular reduction pathways reduce or prevent these activities. It has been proposed that the hypertensive effects of rHb could be due to the protein having too low an affinity for oxygen, causing excessive release of oxygen into the arterioles and vasoconstriction. Alternatively, it has been proposed that NO scavenging by rHb from the vasculature leads to depletion of NO, an increase in intracellular calcium, and muscle constriction. Since the 1980s when researchers started studying rHb, various conjugates and amino acid substitutions have been tested for the ability to reduce issues with stability and toxicity. Through mutagenesis strategies, it has been possible to identify rHb variants with different rates of oxygen binding and release, as well as some that are not associated with increases in blood pressure or mean arterial pressure (MAP). However, more work is needed to identify variants with reduced loss of hemin (a protoporphyrin ring containing chelated iron) and globin denaturation. Work is also underway to lower production costs of rHb variants that are being developed as potential therapeutic products.

1. The table summarizes the difference in blood pressure associated with six variants of rHb along with several parameters in vitro.

rHb	ΔMAP	$k'_{NO, Ox}$	P_{50} (mm HG)	n_{max}	k_{autox}
rHb1	27.5 ± 5.6	57	12	1.8	0.043
rHb2	26.4 ± 1.3	57	37	2.7	0.052
rHb3	22.8 ± 3.6	54	2.8	1.5	0.036
rHb4	18.9 ± 3.2	26	3.9	1.7	0.088
rHb5	11.7 ± 1.5	13	3.3	1.4	0.094
rHb6	6.4 ± 0.9	4	5.4	1.6	0.068

Based on the data in the table, which parameter is most likely to be responsible for the increase in MAP observed for some rHb variants?

a. NO is being scavenged and depleted.
b. Too much oxygen is being released.
c. The affinity for oxygen is too high.
d. rHb is unstable and autoxidation is occurring.

2. In the figure below, the four curves represent rHb variants harboring point mutations and their oxygen-binding curves.

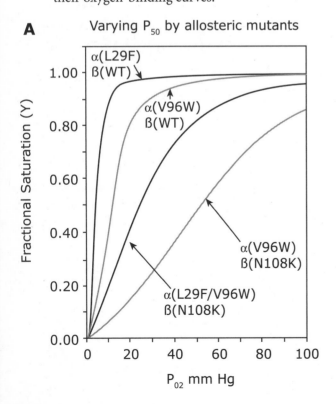

A

Varying P_{50} by allosteric mutants

α(L29F)
β(WT)

α(V96W)
β(WT)

α(V96W)
β(N108K)

α(L29F/V96W)
β(N108K)

Fractional Saturation (Y)

P_{O2} mm Hg

Which curve is most similar to the binding curve of endogenous hemoglobin, and why?

a. The curve for α(L29F)β(WT) because hemoglobin has maximal affinity for oxygen at low and high concentrations
b. The curve for α(V96W)β(WT) because hemoglobin has high affinity for oxygen at low and high concentrations
c. The curve for α(L29F/V96W)β(N108K) because hemoglobin has low affinity for oxygen at low concentrations and high affinity for oxygen at high concentrations
d. The curve for α(V96W)β(N108K) because hemoglobin has low affinity for oxygen at low and high concentrations

3. Engineering a cellular rHBOC involves recombinant DNA technology. What is necessary to make recombinant hemoglobin?

a. Expression of hemoglobin protein in bacteria

b. Knowing the sequence of the hemoglobin gene

c. Knowing the hemoglobin gene's splice donor and acceptor sites

d. Having the crystal structure of hemoglobin protein

4. Which condition would NOT be expected to result in increases in extracellular hemoglobin?

a. Liver cirrhosis

b. Blood transfusion

c. Inflammatory bowel disease

d. Malaria infection

5. Which of the following amino acids does NOT have an isoelectric point (pI) between 5.5 and 6.0?

a. Alanine

b. Glutamic acid

c. Glycine

d. Glutamine

6. Which amino acid would most likely be found on the surface of a protein molecule at physiological pH?

a. Isoleucine

b. Lysine

c. Alanine

d. Proline

7. Which of the following statements about terpenes is NOT true?

a. They are a type of terpenoid.

b. They all contain double bonds.

c. They are all made up of 5-carbon units.

d. They all contain oxygen.

8. How are the plasma membranes of mammalian and bacterial cells similar?

a. They typically contain cholesterol.

b. They have negatively charged lipids on their surfaces.

c. They contain lipids that are involved in signal transduction.

d. They are made up of many different types of phospholipids.

Use the following passage to answer questions 9 through 14.

Under conditions of cell stress, such as exposure to heat, the weak bonds within a protein can be broken, leading to protein misfolding and self-association. When the concentration of misfolded polypeptides becomes high enough, they can form larger aggregates that are very stable because strong bonds occur between the molecules. Many age-related diseases, including Alzheimer's, Parkinson's, and type 2 diabetes, are considered to be the result of protein aggregates, which can eventually cause tissue death. Chaperone molecules bind with high affinity to exposed hydrophobic regions on the surface of misfolded polypeptides and reduce aggregation. However, there is increasing evidence that chaperones do not merely act like sponges that associate with misfolded polypeptides and prevent them from aggregating. Along with a complex of molecules, chaperones can help misfolded substrates unfold and are thus also called unfoldases. Once the substrates are completely unfolded, they can then spontaneously refold into their native conformation. Although chaperones can act on different types of proteins, they unfold them with varying degrees of efficiency. For example, one of the major families of chaperones, which are highly conserved from bacteria to eukaryotes, is called GroEL/GroES. Compared with other chaperones, GroEL/GroES can rapidly convert misfolded rhodanese (rho), a mitochondrial enzyme involved in detoxifying cyanide, into its unfolded form. However, it is unclear in general whether a vast excess of native, properly folded proteins could compete with misfolded substrates for binding to chaperones. Indeed, native proteins are present in a cell at a much higher concentrations relative to misfolded species. Furthermore, if chaperones bind inappropriately to substrates that they are not able to completely unfold, the chaperone molecules may not dissociate rapidly from the partially unfolded species and their activity could get stalled. Another area of question is the role of ATP in the unfolding and refolding of polypeptide substrates. When GroEL/GroES is bound to substrate, ATP hydrolysis leads to conformational changes in GroEL and the release of GroES from the complex. One model is that ATP is not required for the binding of chaperones to misfolded polypeptides but that, at least for some chaperones, ATP hydrolysis is required for the release of the unfolded polypeptide from the chaperone complex so it can refold in solution.

9. The graph below shows the concentration of rhodanese (Rho) that is refolded into its native confirmation in the presence (solid shapes) or absence (open shapes) of an excess concentration of native protein, called MDH. Rhodanese was also incubated with the chaperone GroEL/GroES (LS, ELS) (top four curves) or without (bottom two curves) and with ATP (top two curves) or without (bottom four curves).

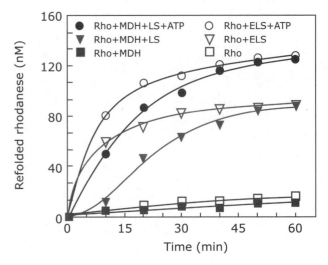

Based on the data presented in the graph, how does native MDH affect the refolding of rhodanese by the chaperone molecules?

a. The refolding is not affected because the chaperones bind MDH and Rho simultaneously.

b. The refolding rate is reduced but the yield of refolding is not changed.

c. The refolding does not occur because MDH stalls the chaperones.

d. The refolding yield is reduced because MDH depletes ATP.

10. Which of the following is NOT a chaperone molecule?
    a. Heat-shock protein (Hsp) 70
    b. SecB
    c. GroEL/GroES
    d. PI3K

11. Which of the following statements is true about the activity of chaperones?
    a. They can act iteratively on many misfolded substrates, one after the other.
    b. They change the chemical composition of misfolded substrates.
    c. They must remain bound to unfolded substrates until they have completely recovered their native conformation.
    d. They require ATP to break apart protein aggregates and unfold misfolded polypeptides.

12. What types of bonds within a protein are likely to be disrupted upon exposure to heat?
    a. covalent bonds
    b. disulfide bonds
    c. hydrogen bonds
    d. carbon bonds

13. Which of these agents does NOT typically denature proteins?
    a. Urea
    b. High pH
    c. Alcohol
    d. HEPES

14. According to the proposed pathway for the action of GroEL/GroES, a single GroEL complex has two subunits consisting of heptameric rings and each ring binds an ATP molecule. How many ADP molecules would be produced when the complex releases an unfolded polypeptide?
    a. 6
    b. 7
    c. 12
    d. 14

15. The digestive enzyme chymotrypsin hydrolyzes nitrophenyl trimethylacetate in a two-step reaction. The initial reaction rate, V0, is 5×10^{-6} M/sec, and the K_M for the reaction is 5.6×10^{-7}. The rate of enzyme-product complex formation is 0.37/sec, and the rate of product release is 1.3×10^{-4}/sec. The total concentration of chymotrypsin is 2×10^{-5} M. What is the maximum rate of the reaction?
    a. 2.6×10^{-9} M/sec
    b. 4.8×10^{-5} M/sec
    c. 1.3×10^{-9} M/sec
    d. 9.5×10^{-6} M/sec

Use the following passage to answer questions 16 through 18.

In the 1950s, doctors demonstrated that methotrexate (MTX) could cause regression of metastatic gestational choriocarcinoma, a highly fatal cancer of the reproductive tract, paving the way to the first chemotherapeutic drug that shrinks solid cancer. Now MTX is used in the treatment of numerous cancers, including breast, lung, osteosarcoma, and leukemia. The original breakthrough arose from the observation that rapidly dividing cells such as tumor cells require folate to make thymine; experts thus reasoned that folate inhibitors could reduce the progression of cancer. MTX is a competitive inhibitor of dihydrofolate reductase (DHFR). By binding to the enzyme, MTX reduces its ability to convert dihydrofolate to folic acid, which is a step in a cellular pathway that is necessary for producing thymine. The association between MTX and DHFR has been shown to involve a complex process and several conformations of the enzyme. However, studies have suggested that MTX acts not only by reducing the level of folic acid; the drug could also directly block the enzyme thymidylate synthase that converts the product of folic acid back to dihydrofolate and as a byproduct generates thymine (in its deoxyribonucleoside 5'-phosphate form, dTMP) from its precursor.

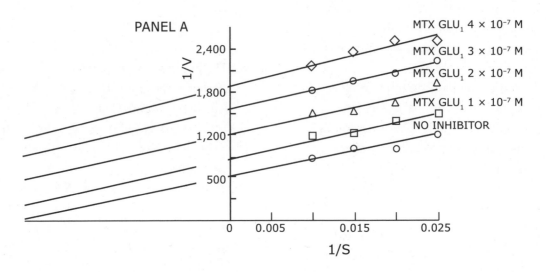

Journal of Biological Chemistry. 1985;260(17):9720–9726. Reprinted with permission.

16. The graph shows a double-reciprocal plot of the rates of inhibition of MTX at different concentrations on thymidylate synthase activity.

Based on the plot, what type of inhibition does MTX exert on thymidylate synthase?

a. Competitive
b. Uncompetitive
c. Mixed (competitive and uncompetitive)
d. Irreversible

17. What is the difference between a competitve and uncompetitive inhibitor of a substrate?
a. A competitive inhibitor does not bind to the enzyme's active site, whereas an uncompetitive inhibitor binds the enzyme.
b. A competitive inhibitor binds near the enzyme's active site, whereas an uncompetitive inhibitor does not bind the enzyme.
c. A competitive inhibitor binds the enzyme's active site, whereas an uncompetitive inhibitor binds outside the enzyme's active site when the enzyme is bound to substrate.
d. A competitive inhibitor binds the enzyme's active site, whereas an uncompetitive inhibitor outside the enzyme's active site when the enzyme is not bound to substrate.

18. Based on the K_D values in the following table, which form of DHFR binds to MTX with the highest affinity?

DHFR variant 1	K_D = 2.2 nM
DHFR variant 2	K_D = 9.5 nM
DHFR variant 3	K_D = 25 nM
DHFR variant 4	K_D = 3×10^{-8} M

    a. Variant 1
    b. Variant 2
    c. Variant 3
    d. Variant 4

19. Which of the following modifications would have the greatest likelihood of improving the yield of polymerase chain reaction (PCR) product?
    a. Increasing the concentration of magnesium (Mg^{2+}) to 1 mM
    b. Reducing the number of cycles
    c. Increasing the concentration of dGTPs and dCTPs
    d. Reducing the denaturation temperature

20. Which chemical modification allows the DNA repair system to distinguish between the DNA template and the newly synthesized strand?
    a. Alkylation
    b. Methylation
    c. Phosphorylation
    d. Histone acetylation

Use the following passage to answer questions 21 through 24.

The fission yeast *Schizosaccharomyces pombe* Rec12 protein, which is the homolog of Spo11 in other organisms, initiates meiotic recombination by creating DNA double-strand breaks (DSBs) and covalently linking to the 5' DNA ends of the break.

This protein-DNA linkage has previously been detected only in mutants such as rad50S, in which break repair is impeded and DSBs accumulate. In the budding yeast *Saccharomyces cerevisiae*, the DSB distribution in a rad50S mutant is markedly different from that in wild-type (RAD50) meiosis, and it was suggested that this might also be true for other organisms. Researchers have shown that linkages between Rec12 and DNA can actually be detected in *Sc. pombe* rad50(+) cells, which are proficient for DSB repair. In fact, genome-wide microarray analysis of Rec12-DNA reveals indistinguishable meiotic DSB distributions in rad50(+) and rad50S strains of *Sc. pombe*, unlike in *Sa. cerevisiae*. These results confirm earlier findings describing the occurrence of widely spaced DSBs primarily in large intergenic regions of DNA and demonstrate the relevance and usefulness of fission yeast studies employing rad50S. The researchers have proposed that the differential behavior of rad50S strains reflects a major difference in DSB regulation between the two species—specifically, the requirement for the Rad50-containing complex for DSB formation in budding yeast but not in fission yeast. Use of rad50S and related mutations may be a useful method for DSB analysis in other species.

21. After DSB and the action of Rec12 (or Spo11), what is the next step that is predicted to occur in DSB repair during meiosis?
    a. The 3' overhang invades the homologous chromosome.
    b. The 5' end and Rec 12 (or Spo 11) invade the homologous chromosome.
    c. The 5' end and Rec 12 (or Spo 11) dissociate, and the 5' end invades the homologous chromosome.
    d. The DSBs are repaired using the homologous chromosomes as the template.

22. The figure is a Southern blot showing the DSB pattern of three strains of *Sc. pombe*, RAD50, rad50S, and a DSB repair double mutant, swi5Δ rhp57Δ, between 0 and 6 hours (h) after the experimental initiation of meiosis.

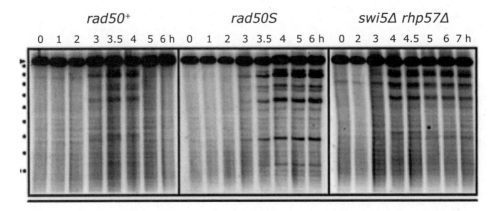

Based on the image, what is the most appropriate conclusion about the DSB patterns in these three strains?

a. DSBs are not observed in rad50+.

b. The three strains have similar DSB patterns and rates of DSB repair.

c. The three strains have similar DSB patterns, but the two mutants do not repair the breaks.

d. The level of DSB intermediates is higher in rad50+ than in the two mutants.

23. Which of the following is NOT a necessary step in Southern blot analysis?
 a. Restriction enzyme treatment of DNA
 b. Amplification of DNA
 c. Separation of DNA by gel electrophoresis
 d. Denaturation of DNA in the gel

24. Detection of DNA by Southern blotting relies on the use of a nucleotide probe that is complementary to sequences in the DNA sample. What prevents RNA from being detected by Southern blotting?
 a. Nucleotide probes do not hybridize to RNA molecules.
 b. RNA cannot be amplified by PCR.
 c. RNA cannot be separated by gel electrophoresis.
 d. DNA can be harvested under conditions that do not allow RNA recovery.

25. How are centromeres and telomeres similar?
 a. Both are required for the distribution of chromosomes during mitosis.
 b. Both are associated with transcriptionally active DNA.
 c. Both are made up of highly repetitive DNA.
 d. Both are conserved in prokaryotic and eukaryotic cells.

Use the following passage to answer questions 26 through 27.

Family and twin studies have suggested that genetic factors could be responsible for 50% to 90% of the variation in bone mineral density (BMD). Therefore, a better understanding of these genes could lead to a more complete understanding of BMD, as well as osteoporosis, which is a condition caused by the loss of BMD and that leads to bone fragility with aging. Population-based case-control studies have identified polymorphisms in many candidate BMD genes. These studies have also highlighted genetic variability between Asian and Caucasian populations in at least five important osteoporosis candidate genes. To take a more extensive look at the genetic variability, researchers investigated single nucleotide polymorphisms (SNPs) in 81 genes associated with osteoporosis by sequencing across exons, splice junctions, and promoter regions. They analyzed these genes among 24 unrelated Korean individuals and compared them to previously reported SNPs in Japanese, Chinese, Caucasian, and African subpopulations. The researchers identified 942 variants, including 888 SNPs, 43 insertion/deletion polymorphisms, and 11 microsatellite markers. They determined whether some of the common SNPs in these subpopulations agree with or deviate from the Hardy-Weinberg principle, which states that genetic variation should remain constant between generations in the absence of factors such as natural selection and nonrandom mating. Further studies of osteoporosis could utilize the polymorphisms identified in this study since they may have important implications for the selection of highly informative SNPs for future association studies.

26. The average F_{IS}, F_{ST}, and F_{IT} values, representing the extent of deviation from the Hardy-Weinberg principle, for the five subpopulations in the study were -0.0121, 0.3366, and 0.3287, respectively. What conclusions can be made about Hardy-Weinberg expectations based on these values?

a. The SNPs in osteoporosis candidate genes are consistent with Hardy-Weinberg expectations both between and within the five subpopulations.

b. The SNPs in osteoporosis candidate genes are consistent with Hardy-Weinberg expectations between the five subpopulations, but the SNPs within the subpopulations differ from Hardy-Weinberg expectations.

c. The SNPs in osteoporosis candidate genes differ from Hardy-Weinberg expectations between the five subpopulations but the SNPs within the subpopulations are consistent with Hardy-Weinberg expectations.

d. The SNPs in osteoporosis candidate genes differ from Hardy-Weinberg expectations both between and within the five subpopulations.

27. In the Korean subpopulation, 36% of individuals are homozygous for a common SNP, whereas 48% do not have the SNP. What percentage of individuals in this subpopulation is heterozygous for the SNP?

a. 8
b. 16
c. 32
d. 42

28. Which of the following is a typical *E. coli* promoter sequence? (N is a nucleotide spacer region.)

a. [AT-rich region]-N-TTGACA-N-TATATG-N-transcription start site

b. [GC-rich region]-N-TTGACA-N-TATATG-N-transcription start site

c. [AT-rich region]-N-TTGACA-N-TATAAT-N-transcription start site

d. [GC-rich region]-N-TTGACA-N-TATAAT-N-transcription start site

29. In the following reaction, what would be the effect of adding more C(s) while maintaining constant pressure?

$$C(s) + CO_2(g) \Leftrightarrow 2CO(g)$$

a. The reaction equilibrium shifts from left to right.

b. The reaction equilibrium shifts from right to left.

c. The reaction equilibrium does not change.

d. The reaction loses equilibrium.

Use the following passage to answer questions 30 through 35.

Changes in the polyol pathway are a leading cause of diabetic complications. The substrate for the pathway is glucose, an essential monosaccharide that falls into the family known as aldoses because it contains a carbonyl group at the end of its carbon chain. In the first step of the pathway, an aldose reductase called ALR2, in the presence of cofactor NADPH, reduces glucose to sorbitol. Then sorbitol dehydrogenase converts sorbitol to fructose along with the reduction of NAD^+. Under nondisease conditions, a low level of glucose enters the polyol pathway because ALR2 has a weak affinity for glucose; most glucose instead goes into the glycolytic pathway. However, under conditions of hyperglycemia, the polyol pathway is activated, leading to the accumulation of sorbitol and a concomitant reduction in NADPH and NAD^+. (The activity of sorbitol dehydrogenase does not increase to deal with the increased levels of sorbitol.) These changes occur primarily in tissues, including the lens, retina, kidney, and peripheral nerves, which do not depend on insulin to take up glucose. The increase in sorbitol, which is not easily cleared from cells, leads to cell swelling and changes in membrane permeability, primarily in the lens. In addition, the drop in NADPH and NAD^+ levels causes an increase in reactive oxygen species (ROS) and oxidative stress. Together, these changes, along with downstream enzymes that respond to changes in the polyol pathway and contribute to oxidative stress and inflammation, precipitate diabetic complications such as cataracts, retinopathy, neuropathy, and atherosclerosis. In the hope of combating some of these complications, researchers have developed a number of ALR inhibitors (ARIs) over the past several decades. Currently, epalrestat is the only ARI that has been approved for clinical use, and it is only approved in Japan, China, and India. The majority of ARIs have not been developed into useful therapies because of their low efficacy and adverse side-effect profiles, which is primarily due to their effects on ALRs that are not involved in the polyol pathway; for instance, ALR1 is active against toxic aldehydes. Consequently, researchers have been designing and testing new ARIs derived from a cyclical molecule called quinoxaline. To evaluate these derivatives' efficacy, the researchers have tested their ability to inhibit ALR2 based on their IC50 values. IC50 corresponds to the drug concentration that is required to inhibit 50% of the activity of an enzyme. However, it has been proposed that for a drug to effectively prevent and reduce diabetic complications, it may have to suppress oxidative stress as well as reduce ALR activity. As a result, researchers are working to develop drugs that also have anti-oxidative properties. Compounds that exhibit both of these properties would be pursued for their ability to constitute important new multifunctional ARIs.

Glucose

Fructose

30. The polyol pathway metabolizes glucose into fructose. Based on their chemical structures, to which monosaccharide families do glucose and fructose belong?

   a. Glucose is an aldose and fructose is a hexose.

   b. Glucose is an aldose and fructose is a ketose.

   c. Glucose is a ketose and fructose is an aldose.

   d. They are both aldoses.

31. Which of the following monosaccharides is essential for humans and can be obtained at high levels from diet?

   a. Glucose

   b. Galactose

   c. Fructose

   d. Fucose

32. Which cell type uses insulin to help take up glucose?

   a. Lens

   b. Adipose

   c. Kidney

   d. Nerves

33. Based on the provided chemical structure, quinoxaline is an analog of what type of hydrocarbon?

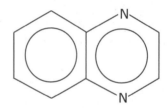

   a. Cyclohexane

   b. Benzene

   c. Anthracene

   d. Naphthalene

34. Based on the table, which compound derived from quinoxaline would be predicted to be the most effective treatment for diabetic complications and carries the lowest risk of adverse side effect?

COMPOUND	IC$_{50}$ FOR ALR2	IC$_{50}$ FOR ALR1
3	0.498	6.9
6	0.065	29.8
8	0.412	24.3
13	0.067	6.4

    a. Compound 3
    b. Compound 6
    c. Compound 8
    d. Compound 13

35. To determine if quinoxaline-derived compounds are potent antioxidants, researchers exposed them to DPPH, which is a free radical that loses its purple color when it accepts hydrogen. Using this assay, what method could be used to quantitatively measure the antioxidative activities of the compounds?
    a. Spectrophotometry
    b. Enzyme digest
    c. Gel electrophoresis
    d. Electron microscopy

Use the following passage to answer questions 36 through 39.

Noncoding RNA molecules have the potential to play important roles both in the development and treatment of cancer. Of the many classes of noncoding RNA molecules, two types are dysregulated in hepatocellular carcinoma (HCC) and various other types of cancer: microRNAs (miRNAs) and long noncoding RNAs (lncRNAs). MiRNAs are short (21 to 23 nucleotides) single-stranded RNAs that are processed from longer precursor miRNAs and that are found in most organisms. This RNA species usually binds to messenger RNAs (mRNAs) that have regions of near-perfect complementarity, which represses translation or, in some cases, leads to cleavage of the mRNa. LncRNAs, on the other hand, are generally defined as RNA molecules that are longer than 200 nucleotides. They often resemble mRNA molecules because of features such as being capped and polyadenylated, and they are actually more abundant than protein-coding RNAs in the cell. Although lncRNAs were originally thought of as transcriptional noise or artifacts of cloning, recent studies suggest that they play a number of regulatory roles in gene expression and in localization of proteins and subcellular structures; lncRNAs are also small RNA precursors. In the case of both miRNAs and lncRNAs, changes in expression levels have been associated with HCC survival and response to treatment. For example, overexpression of an lncRNA called HOTTIP may be responsible for chemoresistance. Decreased expression of a miRNA called miR26 has been associated with shorter survival but also superior response to interferon therapy for hepatitis C virus (HCV), whereas decreased expression of miR122 has also been linked with poor progression in patients with HCC. The differential expression of noncoding RNA in HCCs suggests that these molecules could serve as biomarkers if the differential expression can be shown more consistently among studies than it has been to date. There is particular need for noninvasive biomarkers that allow detection of early HCC. Several properties of RNAs make them attractive clinical tools, including the fact that they can be detected in patient sera, they are stable, and sensitive detection methods are available, such as microarray and polymerase chain reaction. On the therapeutic side, noncoding RNAs have become new molecular targets for HCC drugs. The leading drug candidate is called Miravirsen, and it inhibits miR122, which is required for replication of HCV. Miravirsen is currently in phase II clinical trials. Another class of noncoding RNAs, called short interfering RNAs (siRNAs), is also being developed as a potential HCC therapeutic. Although siRNAs are not normally expressed in human cells, the potent ability of these 22-nucleotide molecules to bind and degrade mRNAs with complementary sequence makes them highly valuable tools for targeting cellular proteins. Similar to miRNAs, siRNAs can be processed from a double-stranded RNA molecule by a cellular protein called Dicer. One siRNA-based treatment for primary as well as metastatic liver cancer destroys the RNAs encoding kinesin spindle protein and vascular endothelial growth factor. Currently, this drug has been found to be safe in phase I clinical trials. Furthermore, siRNAs could be developed that target lncRNAs that are critical for the development of progression of HCC. As more clinical studies are conducted on these novel drug candidates, several obstacles will need to be overcome. Major challenges include the off-target effects of short noncoding RNAs: both miRNA and siRNA species have been reported to bind mRNAs with imperfect complementarity and cause their translational repression. In addition, the clinical application of noncoding RNAs will require improved chemical formulations that ensure their delivery to appropriate tissues in the body.

36. How are miRNAs and siRNAs different from each other?
   a. MiRNAs are generally longer than siRNAs.
   b. MiRNAs block translation, whereas siRNAs degrade mRNAs.
   c. MiRNAs are endogenously expressed in humans, whereas siRNAs are exogenously expressed.
   d. MiRNAs do not undergo processing in cells, whereas siRNAs are processed through the Dicer pathway.

37. Which of the following features would lncRNAs NOT be expected to have?
   a. 5'-capping
   b. Acetylation
   c. Polyadenylation
   d. Splice donor and acceptor sites

38. What types of noncoding RNA species would be predicted to have the following sequences (where N_x represents x number of nucleotides)?

   Sequence 1 uggagugugacaaugguguuug
   Sequence 2 cccuuccuuuaucccagugggggcccaga cccgcgcaaccaggcggggaggggaggugggc (N_{3660}) ggauaguuuuuccaccuuugcccgauacaauuu aaaaaaaaaaa
   a. Sequence 1 is an miRNA; sequence 2 is an lncRNA.
   b. Sequence 1 is an lncRNA; sequence 2 is an miRNA.
   c. Sequence 1 is an lncRNA; sequence 2 is an siRNA.
   d. Both sequences are miRNAs.

39. Which of the following properties would need to be improved to use noncoding RNA as diagnostic markers?

 a. Stability

 b. Ability to detect them in sera

 c. Ability to amplify them to improve detection sensitivity

 d. Reliable changes in expression levels in patients with HCC

40. Some species of coldwater fish have proteins in their blood that can lower the blood's freezing point. If the concentration of these so-called antifreeze proteins in the blood is 4×10^{-3} m_c, what is the freezing point depression?

 a. 0.002 K

 b. 0.007 K

 c. 1.15 K

 d. 3.16 K

Use the following passage to answer questions 41 through 44.

Although common neurological diseases, such as Alzheimer's, Parkinson's, and amyotrophic lateral sclerosis (ALS), have distinct symptoms and molecular mechanisms, they share one important feature: they all involve the death of neuronal cells. In the case of Alzheimer's, cell death occurs in the brain and is nonspecific, whereas with Parkinson's and ALS, it is limited to dopaminergic neurons and motor neurons, respectively. Nevertheless, because the pathologies of these diseases all lead to the destruction of nerve cells, stem cell–based regeneration has the potential to be effective against all of them. Stem cells are defined by two important properties: their potential to proliferate and to differentiate into multiple cell types. They can be derived from embryonic tissue (embryonic stem cells [ESCs]) and fetal tissue (fetal stem cells [FSCs]). However, ESCs and FCSs face a number of complications, particularly ethical concerns and questions about tumor formation and immune rejection after transplantation. In 2006, researchers made a potential breakthrough in stem cell therapy when they demonstrated that c-Myc, Sox2, Oct4, and Klf4 could reprogram somatic cells into a state of pluripotency. Nevertheless, the induction of pluripotency is an inefficient process, and the requirement to overexpress c-Myc and the other factors similarly raised concerns about tumor formation as a potential adverse side effect. An alternative source of stem cells is self-renewing cells that reside in the epithelial lining of skin, stomach, intestine, and other tissues and that help replenish the tissue after exposure to environmental insults. These cells are referred to as adult stem cells (ASCs), and they are multipotent, meaning that they can differentiate into all of the cell types of their resident tissue. ASCs do not present the same ethical dilemma as ESCs and FSCs and may solve concerns of immune rejection if autologous transplants are used. As a result, much work has been devoted to characterizing the biomarkers found on the surface of ASCs to understand and isolate these cell populations. Yet ASCs still present challenges, such as difficulty harvesting, poor proliferation, and limited differentiation. One type of ASCs, mesenchymal stem cells (MSCs), has the advantage of being relatively easy to isolate from samples such as the spinal fluid or umbilical cord blood, and they also expand well in tissue culture. In addition, it has been demonstrated that MSCs not only differentiate into bone, cartilage, and adipocyte cells but could also give rise to a variety of other cell types, including neurons. Once in the body, the localization of MSCs could rely on cytokines and growth factors, such as platelet-derived growth factor, that mediate cell migration. In one study, intravenous administration of spinal fluid–derived MSCs was found to improve symptoms in patients following a stroke. However, numerous studies have raised doubt about whether the beneficial effects of MSCs in the treatment of neurological diseases are due to paracrine effects of these cells rather than their ability to directly lead to the regeneration of neuronal cells, which is required for functional recovery from neuronal diseases. For this reason, adult neural stem cells (NSCs), which exhibit both paracrine and direct differentiation effects, are also being pursued in the development of clinical therapies. The drawbacks with NSCs, however, are the difficulty of harvesting them from the unique microenvironment of the subventricular and subgranular zones in the brain and their less robust proliferation capacity. Despite the challenges, researchers have had success isolating very small brain samples for the isolation of NSCs. Although studies are in preclinical and early clinical trials, stem cell–based therapy seems to hold the greatest potential against diseases such as stroke, Parkinson's, and ALS. Unfortunately, this therapy may not hold great promise for patients with Alzheimer's because the widespread neuronal death in the brain makes harvesting cells for NSC difficult and the disease process that leads to neuronal cell destruction in the first place could quickly destroy transplanted cells.

41. What type of cellular protein induces pluripotency in somatic cells?
   a. Cell cycle proteins
   b. Kinases
   c. Transcription factors
   d. Transmembrane proteins

42. Which type of stem cell is the best choice for the treatment of neurological diseases?
   a. ESCs
   b. FSCs
   c. Induced pluripotent stem cells
   d. ASCs

43. Which of the following characteristics would NOT be essential for the validation of MSC cells in tissue culture?
   a. They must adhere to the plastic surface of Petri dishes.
   b. They must express a specific subset of markers on their surface.
   c. They must show the capacity to differentiate into osteoblasts, adipocytes, and chrondoblasts.
   d. They must be dependent on a specific subset of growth factors for proliferation.

44. Which of the following would NOT be a predicted mechanism by which MSCs lead to improvements in neurological symptoms in patients?
   a. Secretion of growth factors
   b. Secretion of pluripotency-inducing factors
   c. Release of anti-apoptotic factors
   d. Secretion of cytokines

Use the following passage to answer questions 45 through 47.

Compared with their eukaryotic counterparts, bacteria are small and have simple structures. Their genomes are a mere 1 to 5 million nucleotides, compared with the 12 million of yeast and 3 billion of humans. Despite their diminutive size, a subset of these organisms can cause devastating disease in humans, animals, and plants. When a bacterial infection is suspected in a clinical setting, the Gram stain is often the first test that is performed, which allows classification of the bacteria as either Gram-positive or Gram-negative. Gram-positive bacteria, such as *Staphylococci*, possess a single membrane and a cell wall that is thick and is composed of cross-linked peptidoglycan. Bacteria in this group retain the violet dye used in the Gram stain procedure. Gram-negative bacteria, such as *Salmonella*, possess two membranes that are separated from each other by a periplasmic space. The cell wall is located in this space in Gram-negative bacteria, and it is thinner than in Gram-positive bacteria; as a result, Gram-negative bacteria cannot retain the violet dye used in Gram staining. Bacteria can be also be classified based on their shape: spheres (cocci), such as *Streptococcus*; rods (bacilli), such as *E. coli*; and spiral cells (spirochetes). However, many bacteria have similar shapes within the Gram-positive and Gram-negative categories. Another way to distinguish between different bacteria is based on the proteins on the cell surface. Many bacteria have helical flagella on their surface that they use for propulsion, or pili spikes that allow them to adhere to host tissue. There are also more specific tests. For example, the Lancefield system groups *Streptococci* (groups A–H, K–M, O–V) based on the carbohydrate groups on their surface, which can be detected using antibody-based tests. Some tests rely on enzymatic activity. The catalase test differentiates aerobic and anaerobic bacteria because only the former express high levels of the catalase enzyme, which converts hydrogen peroxide to hydrogen and oxygen. The presence of catalase can be detected in this test because the bacteria produce bubbles in the presence of hydrogen peroxide. Other enzyme tests involve growing the bacteria on specialized agar plates. For example, lactose-fermenting enteric bacteria, including *E. coli* and *Klebsiella*, can be identified on MacConkey agar. These bacteria ferment the lactose in the agar, causing the pH of the lactose to change and the agar to undergo an easily perceptible change in color.

Staphylococcus aureus can be distinguished from other *Staphylococci* species because it has coagulase activity, which results in hemolysis of red blood cells on a blood agar plate. These and a panel of other tests are routinely performed in clinical microbiology labs, either by hand or automated machines, to identify organisms from patient samples.

45. Which set of test results would lead to the positive identification of *Staphylococcus aureus* in a patient sample?
   a. Gram-positive, cocci-shaped, catalase-positive, coagulase-positive
   b. Gram-positive, cocci-shaped, catalase-negative, coagulase-positive
   c. Gram-positive, rod-shaped, catalase-positive, coagulase-positive
   d. Gram-negative, cocci-shaped, catalase-positive, coagulase-positive

46. Based on the image, what types of bacteria could be depicted?

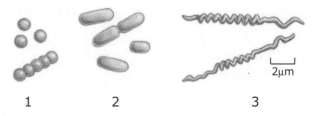

http://www.ncbi.nlm.nih.gov/books/NBK26917/.

   a. 1, *Streptococcus pyogenes*; 2, *Staphylococcus aureus*; 3, *Borrelia burgdorferi*
   b. 1, *Escherichia coli*; 2, *Streptococcus pyogenes*; 3, *Borrelia burgdorferi*
   c. 1, *Escherichia coli*; 2, *Streptococcus pyogenes*; 3, *Treponema pallidum*
   d. 1, *Streptococcus pyogenes*; 2, *Escherichia coli*; 3, *Treponema pallidum*

47. Based on the image, what type of bacteria could have this type of cell membrane and wall?

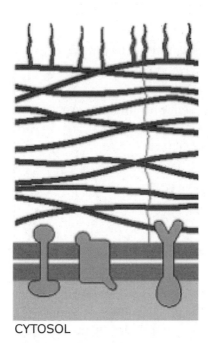

CYTOSOL

http://www.ncbi.nlm.nih.gov/books/NBK26917/.

    a. *Salmonella bongori*
    b. *Escherichia coli*
    c. *Bacillus anthracis*
    d. *Neisseria meningitidis*

48. Based on the table, which of the gases would have the highest concentration in water at 25°C with the pressure of 1 atm?

GAS	k_h (atm/M) AT 25°C
He	2.7×10^3
N_2	1.6×10^3
O_2	7.8×10^2
CO_2	29

    a. He
    b. N_2
    c. O_2
    d. CO_2

Use the following passage to answer questions 49 through 52.

Energy homeostasis is tightly controlled by the central nervous system (CNS), and in particular a region of the brain called the hypothalamus, in conjunction with peripheral signals that convey information to the CNS. When the process becomes imbalanced, it can lead to metabolic disorders such as obesity, as well as cardiovascular diseases, hypertension, stroke, and type 2 diabetes. The neuronal circuit in the hypothalamus that is most critical for energy homeostasis is called the melanocortin system. This system is made up of three neuronal populations: neurons that express agouti-related peptide (AgRP) and the neuropeptide Y (NPY) and neurons that express proopiomelanocortin, both of which are located in the hypothalamic arcuate nucleus, and neurons that express the melanocortin 4 receptor (MC4R), located in the hypothalamic paraventricular nucleus. POMC neurons are anorexigenic because, by activating MC4R, they reduce food intake and increase energy expenditure. On the other hand, AgRP/NPY neurons are orexigenic because they antagonize the activity of POMC. POMC is a large polypeptide hormone that is processed by proteases that cleave in between basic residues to produce nine proteins. Of these proteins, α-MSH is a well-known anorexigenic molecule that exerts its effect by binding and activating melanocortin receptors. A number of peripheral hormones also regulate the melanocortin neurons, including leptin, insulin, ghrelin, glucocorticoids, and thyroid hormones. In particular, the leptin hormone, which is produced by adipocytes, has received a lot of attention for its potential to combat obesity. Mice that carry two defective variants of the gene encoding leptin have abnormal growth, have an unbridled appetite, and become obese. Furthermore, the receptors for leptin, unlike the receptors for hormones such as insulin, are primarily expressed in the brain in regions that control eating behavior, namely the hypothalamic arcuate nucleus and the hypothalamic paraventricular nucleus. Binding of leptin to its receptor, Ob-Rb, activates a JAK-STAT signaling pathway that leads to the activation of expression of the POMC gene and thus exerts anorexigenic effects. Despite the involvement of leptin in food intake, however, injection of the hormone is not associated with weight reduction. This finding suggests that steps in energy homeostasis that are downstream of leptin expression, as well as other factors, also play key roles in obesity. The insulin hormone, produced by β-pancreatic cells, has receptors in many organs, including the hypothalamus. Similar to leptin, insulin signals for the increased production of POMC; insulin receptors in NPY neurons decrease the production of the orexigenic NPY. Unlike leptin and insulin, ghrelin stimulates orexigenic neurons. Also in contrast to leptin and insulin, this hormone produced by endocrine cells in the stomach acts on a short time scale and is responsible for rapid feelings of sharp hunger. In addition to these and other hormones, the melanocortin system is regulated by nutrients such as glucose, lipids, and amino acids. The interplay of neuroendocrine mediators has evolved to control food intake and metabolism, to prevent starvation, and to avoid harmful obesity.

49. What would be the predicted effect of mutations that disrupt the POMC gene?
   a. Decreased fat accumulation
   b. Increased fat accumulation
   c. Upregulation of α-MSH
   d. Activation of MC4R neurons

50. Between which two amino acids would a POMC protease cleave?
   a. Arg-Gln
   b. Asp-His
   c. Arg-Lys
   d. Lys-Glu

51. Following binding of leptin to Ob-Rb, what is the next step in the signaling pathway?
   a. The POMC gene is upregulated.
   b. The receptor molecules dimerize.
   c. The intracellular region of the receptor is phosphorylated.
   d. The STAT signaling molecule is phosphorylated.

52. Which hormones follow the patterns shown in the graphs below?

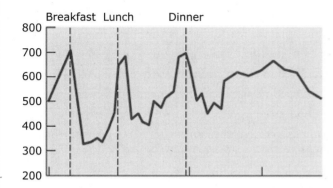

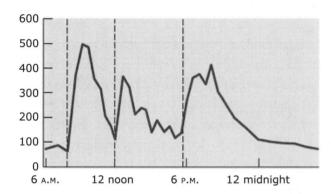

a. The top graph is insulin; the bottom graph is leptin.

b. The top graph is leptin; the bottom graph is insulin.

c. The top graph is insulin; the bottom graph is ghrelin.

d. The top graph is ghrelin; the bottom graph is insulin.

53. Based on the graph, which of the following is NOT true about the role of natural killer (NK) cells in controlling viral infection?

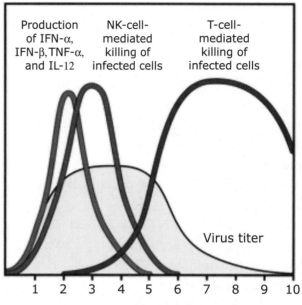

a. They are activated in response to interferon molecules and some cytokines.

b. They are part of the adaptive immune response to viruses, along with T-cells.

c. Their levels decline as T-cells start to be produced.

d. They help control virus replication in the initial days of infection.

54. Which class of immunoglobulin is the first to be made after B-cell activation?

a. IgA

b. IgE

c. IgG

d. IgM

Use the following passage to answer questions 55 through 57.

The typical route of absorption of orally administered drugs is via intestinal cells called enterocytes. Drugs are transported across these cells and in most cases then diffuse into the portal vein, which brings blood from the intestines to the liver. Absorption through this route, however, involves first-pass metabolism through the liver, which significantly reduces the concentration of the drug that makes it into systemic blood. An alternative route that avoids this effect is for drugs to enter lymphatic vessels after transport across enterocytes. There is a dense layer of blood and lymphatic vessels underlying enterocytes of the gastrointestinal tract, yet because of the higher flow rate of portal blood, the majority of compounds take this route. However, there are drug properties that can encourage lymphatic drug uptake. For example, the diffusion of drug molecules across the blood vessel endothelium can get blocked, and as a result intestinal lymph transport is favored because lymphatic capillaries are more permeable than blood capillaries. In addition, the association of drug compounds with lipoproteins in enterocytes not only facilitates their transport through these cells but also preferentially releases them into lymphatic vessels because they are too big to diffuse into blood vessels. As a result, lipophilic drugs, such as cyclosporine, halofantrine, and testosterone derivatives, have lymphatic transport, which studies have shown contribute to their bioavailability. In contrast, hydrophilic drugs, such as caffeine and salicylic acid, are primarily taken up by blood vessels. The type of lipid determines the lipophilicity of the compound: fatty acid chains with more than 14 carbons are more lipophilic than shorter chains, and unsaturated fatty acids are more likely to undergo lymphatic transport than saturated

fatty acids. Many drugs have been modified with these types of lipids to improve bioavailability. For example, a study of the HIV drug didanosine conjugated the compound to triglycerides. Even though lipid modifications have been found to adversely affect activity for other drugs, the study found that triglyceride derivatives of didanosine did not become significantly more toxic to peripheral blood mononuclear cells in culture, based on CD_{50} values, which is the concentration of drug at which half of the cells die. In addition, the derivates were similar to unmodified didanosine in their effective dose, or ED_{50} values, which in this case is the concentration of drug that inhibits viral reverse transcriptase activity. In addition to boosting better bioavailability, HIV drugs that have increased lymphatic transport could be especially effective against this virus because it has been suggested that the gut lymphatic system is critical in the development of infection. Several other viruses are also thought to spread through the lymphatic network, such as hepatitis B, hepatitis C, and severe acute respiratory syndrome. This network is also the primary route for transport of B and T cells, as well as metastasis of solid tumors. Thus, immunomodulatory compounds and anticancer drugs could also be effective if they were absorbed lymphatically.

55. Which of these lipids would be expected to most improve lymphatic uptake in the gut when conjugated to a drug compound?
  a. choline
  b. glycerol
  c. palmitic acid
  d. phosphatidylcholine

56. What drug compound property would NOT be expected to improve its bioavailability?
   a. Molecular weight increase
   b. Molecular weight decrease
   c. Colloidal material design
   d. Hydrophilicity

57. Based on the data in the table, which compound would be expected to be the most toxic?

COMPOUND	ED_{50} (μM)	CD_{50} (μM)
didanosine	3.2	11.0
didanosine-derivative 1	1.5	9.4
didanosine-derivative 2	7.2	51.2
didanosine-derivative 3	26.2	12.7

   a. didanosine
   b. didanosine-derivative 1
   c. didanosine-derivative 2
   d. didanosine-derivative 3

58. In what way are the molecular motor proteins kinesin and dynein similar to each other?
   a. Both are associated with microtubules.
   b. Both are involved in fast axonal transport.
   c. Both are inhibited by the ATP analog AMP-PNP.
   d. Both conduct primarily retrograde axonal transport.

59. The FDA recently approved a laboratory test for determining a patient's risk of developing acute kidney injury (AKI). In this test, increases in urinary levels of tissue inhibitor of metalloproteinase 2 (TIMP-2) and insulin-like growth factor binding protein 7 (IGFBP-7) are predictive of AKI. Based on the plot, where light gray bars represent patients with AKI based on Kidney Disease: Improving Global Outcomes classification and the dark gray bars represent patients without AKI, what can be concluded about this new test's usefulness in patients pre-surgery (1), immediately after surgery (2), 4 hours after surgery (3), and the first postoperative morning (4)?

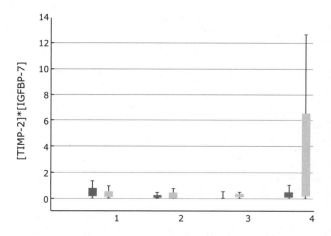

Critical Care. 2015;19:3. Reprinted with permission.

   a. It can determine the risk of AKI before and after surgery.
   b. It can predict preoperatively who will develop AKI on the first postoperative day.
   c. It can distinguish between patients with and without AKI on the first postoperative day.
   d. It is not a precise predictor of AKI risk either before or after surgery.

Part 2: Chemical and Physical Foundations of Biological Systems

59 Questions
95 Minutes

1. The average total lung capacity of an adult human male is 6.0 L of air at a body temperature of 310 K and atmospheric pressure. Given that air is 78.1% nitrogen, how many nitrogen molecules would be present in the lungs of an adult human male when filled to capacity with air?

   a. 8.26×10^{22} molecules N_2
   b. 1.11×10^{23} molecules N_2
   c. 1.42×10^{23} molecules N_2
   d. 1.84×10^{23} molecules N_2

2. What is the pH of a solution of 0.805 M benzoic acid and 0.0800 M potassium benzoate if its K_a value is 6.28×10^{-5}?

   a. 3.20
   b. 4.50
   c. 5.30
   d. 6.10

3. When 5.00 mL of ethanol (MW = 46.1 g/mol) was burned in an excess of oxygen gas (MW = 32.0 g/mol), 1.10 mL of water (MW = 18.0 g/mol) was collected. The density of ethanol is 0.789 g/mL, and the density of water is 1.00 g/mL. What is the percent yield for this reaction?

   a. 18.8%
   b. 24.3%
   c. 35.7%
   d. 71.4%

Questions 4 through 7 are based on the following passage.

The homodimeric DNA-binding protein Ssh10b, from *Sulfolobus shibattae*, is conserved in the majority of currently sequenced thermophilic and hyperthermophilic archaeal genomes. Denaturation of Ssh10b by urea, a chaotropic agent, was tested at five different pH values (3, 5, 7, 9, and 10) and eight different NaCl salt concentrations (0 M [black squares], 0.01 M [open squares], 0.02 M [black circles], 0.05 M [open circles], 0.1 M [black triangles], 0.2 [open triangles], 0.5 M [inverted black triangles], and 1 M [inverted open triangles]). The results are shown in Figure 1.

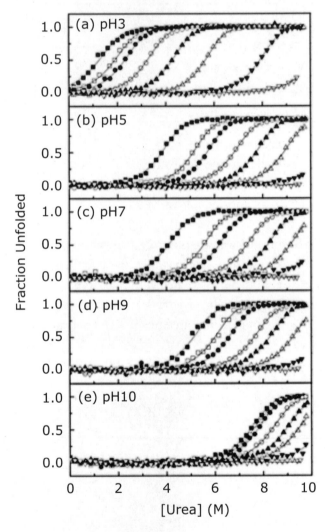

Figure 1. The effects of pH and salt concentration on urea-induced Ssh10b unfolding at 25° C.
Yong-Jin Mao, Xiang-Rong Sheng, Xian-Ming Pan, © 2007 Mao et al; licensee BioMed Central Ltd. This image is available from http://www.biomedcentral.com/1471-2091/8/28.

The structure of urea is shown in Figure 2.

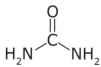

Figure 2. The structure of urea.

4. What is the most likely mode of protein denaturation by urea, based on its structure?
   a. Disruption of crosslink bonds between monomers
   b. Breakage of disulfide bonds within the tertiary structure of the protein
   c. Disruption of the hydrogen-bonding network in the protein
   d. Promotion of peptide bond hydrolysis to break the amino acid chain

5. Based on the results obtained, what effect do the tested salt concentrations have on protein stability?
   a. At low pH, increased salt concentration results in increased protein stability, but at high pH, protein stability is independent of salt concentration.
   b. At high pH, increased salt concentration results in increased protein stability, but at low pH, protein stability is independent of salt concentration.
   c. At the tested pH, increased salt concentration consistently decreases protein stability.
   d. At the tested pH, increased salt concentration consistently increases protein stability.

6. The pK_a values for four buffers at room temperature are shown in the table.

BUFFER	pK_a
Glycine-HCl	2.4
Sodium acetate	4.8
HEPES	7.6
Ammonium acetate	4.76, 9.24

Which buffer would be most appropriate for obtaining the denaturation curves displayed in Figure 1, panel c?

   a. Glycine-HCl
   b. Sodium acetate
   c. HEPES
   d. Ammonium acetate

7. In the presence of salt, what effect does pH have on the unfolding free energy (ΔG) of Ssh10b?
   a. The unfolding ΔG increases as pH increases.
   b. The unfolding ΔG increases as pH decreases.
   c. The unfolding ΔG increases at low pH and decreases at high pH.
   d. The unfolding ΔG decreases at low pH and increases at high pH.

Questions 8 through 11 are based on the following information.

A horizontal spring is bolted to a wall on one end and is attached to a box on the other end (Figure 1). At rest, the distance between the wall and the box is 0.5 meters. The box itself has a mass of 1.0 kg, and the spring constant is 5.0 N/m.

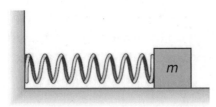

Figure 1. A box is attached to a horizontal spring.

Several different weights, of mass m, were added to the box to change its overall mass. For each trial, the box was moved 0.75 meters away from the wall, the spring's full extension. All motion is frictionless.

8. The number of oscillation cycles that the spring completes in a given time frame is called the
   a. velocity.
   b. acceleration.
   c. period.
   d. frequency.

9. As more mass, m, is added to the box, how does the potential energy of the box at the end of the extended spring change?
   a. The potential energy of the box increases as m increases.
   b. The potential energy of the box decreases as m increases.
   c. The potential energy of the box stays the same as m increases.
   d. The potential energy of the box increases or decreases based on the rate of change of the spring constant.

10. For the spring system described in Figure 1, what is the potential energy when the spring is fully extended and no mass m is added?
   a. 0.63 J
   b. 1.4 J
   c. 2.5 J
   d. 3.1 J

11. The kinetic energy of the box is increasing. Therefore, the box must be
   a. moving toward equilibrium.
   b. moving away from equilibrium.
   c. moving to the left.
   d. moving to the right.

Questions 12 through 15 are based on the following information.

A voltaic cell is set up to study the reaction below, with two vessels connected by a salt bridge and wire at 25°C:

$$MnO_4^- + 3VO^{2+} + H_2O \rightarrow MnO_2 + 6H^+ + 3VO_2^+$$

The following table provides standard reduction potentials at 25°C for the two relevant half-reactions:

HALF-REACTION	STANDARD REDUCTION POTENTIAL (V)
$MnO_4^- + 4H^+ + 3e^- \rightarrow MnO_2 + 2H_2O$	+1.68
$VO_2^+ + 2H^+ + e^- \rightarrow VO^{2+} + H_2O$	+1.00

12. In a voltaic cell like the one described, a reduction reaction occurs at
   a. the anode.
   b. the cathode.
   c. both the anode and the cathode.
   d. neither the anode nor the cathode.

13. In the reaction described, which element is being oxidized over the course of the reaction of interest?
   a. H
   b. Mn
   c. O
   d. V

14. What is the VSEPR shape of the Mn-containing reactant species?
   a. Square planar
   b. Tetrahedral
   c. Linear
   d. Seesaw

$$O = Mn - O^-$$

with O double-bonded above and below the Mn.

There are four possible resonance structures, with the single bond on each of the four oxygens, but for the purposes of VSEPR shapes, these resonance structures are not particularly important. What is important is that there are no lone pairs on the Mn atom that will influence the shape of the molecule. There are four ligands on Mn, and there are no lone pairs on the central atom. Therefore, the shape of the molecule is tetrahedral. There are no lone pairs on Mn that would cause the square planar shape. This shape is usually observed when there are four ligands and two lone pairs on the central atom. Linear configurations most commonly occur in molecules with two ligands on the central atom. And Seesaw configurations commonly occur when there are four ligands and two lone electron pairs on a central atom. Since there are four ligands and no lone pairs on Mn in permanganate, this is not the correct shape.

15. Given that Faraday's constant is 96,485 C/mol, what is the value of $\Delta G°$ for the reaction of interest?

  a. −65.7 kJ

  b. −197 kJ

  c. 127 kJ

  d. 382 kJ

Questions 16 through 19 are based on the following passage.

Metabolic labeling of proteins can be used for insight into their turnover rates. Such labeling was used to follow the turnover of specific proteins from the single-celled green algae *Chlamydomonas reinhardtii*. To accomplish this labeling for proteins in the algae, growth medium was prepared with standard Tris-acetate-phosphate (TAP) medium in which nitrogen-containing components of the media had their nitrogen atoms replaced with ^{14}N, allowing for normal algal cell growth. By mass spectrometry, it was determined that ^{15}N was incorporated into 13 amino acids at approximately 98% labeling efficiency. The ^{14}N- and ^{15}N-labeled crude algal protein extracts were mixed with detergent-like sodium dodecyl sulfate and separated by size and charge using SDS-PAGE. The 55-kDa SDS-PAGE bands from the crude extracts were digested using trypsin, and 27 proteins were identified by LC-MS/MS. Five of these proteins, present in both the labeled and unlabeled samples, exhibited peptide sequence confidence levels higher than 95% and protein sequence coverage higher than 25%. After the newly synthesized ^{15}N-labeled free amino acids and proteins reached maximal ^{15}N incorporation, turnover rates were determined after the cells were transferred into unlabeled TAP medium. Turnover rates were measured in terms of fractional abundance (R_t), with ^{14}N and ^{15}N levels quantified using the peak magnitude on the MS/MS spectrum, for each peptide of three proteins of interest from the extracts (Figure 1).

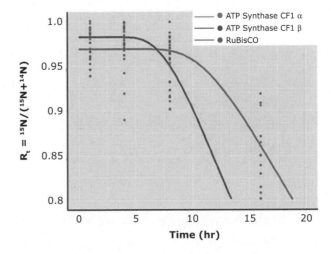

Figure 1. Protein turnovers for the initial 20 hours.
Source: Sauer et al. Metabolic labeling with stable isotope nitrogen (15N) to follow amino acid and protein turnover of three plastid proteins in *Chalamydomonas reinhardtii*. *Proteome Science.* 2014; 12:14.

16. A feature of algal cells such as *Chlamydomonas reinhardtii* cells that might increase the difficulty of experimental cell lysis is

  a. the presence of membrane-bound organelles.

  b. the presence of a chitin-based cell wall.

  c. the presence of a cellulose-based cell wall.

  d. the absence of a nucleus.

17. What is the difference in mass between a fully labeled and unlabeled free asparagine amino acid, based on the labeling method described in the passage?

  a. 1 amu

  b. 2 amu

  c. 3 amu

  d. 4 amu

18. Why would a significant increase in R_t never be observed in Figure 1?

    a. R_t measures the absolute quantity of labeled free amino acids and proteins in labeled media, so additional labeling will occur from media molecules that are already being detected.

    b. R_t measures the fraction of total free amino acids and proteins that are labeled in labeled media, so additional labeling will occur from media molecules that are already being detected.

    c. R_t measures the absolute quantity of labeled free amino acids and proteins after transfer to the unlabeled media, so no additional detection of isotope labels should occur.

    d. R_t measures the fraction of total free amino acids and proteins that are labeled after transfer to the unlabeled media, so no additional detection of isotope labels should occur.

19. During which experimental procedure does denaturation of the proteins of interest first occur?

    a. Cell growth in ^{15}N-labeled TAP media

    b. SDS-PAGE

    c. Trypsin digestion

    d. LC-MS/MS

Questions 20 through 23 are based on the following passage.

Capillaries are fine, branching blood vessels that connect arteriole and venule vessels (Figure 1; page 54). They work as networks called capillary beds and allow for fluid, nutrient, and waste exchange between the blood and body tissues. The porous capillary walls allow for diffusion of water and small solutes, while larger biomolecules like proteins cannot pass through. At the arteriole end, fluid moves from the vessel to the body tissue, while at the venule end, fluid, gas, and wastes enter the capillary from the body tissue. In the central portion of the capillary network, fluid passes equally between the capillary and body tissues, and general gas, nutrient, and waste exchange takes place. In particular, fluid exchange is controlled by hydrostatic and osmotic pressure.

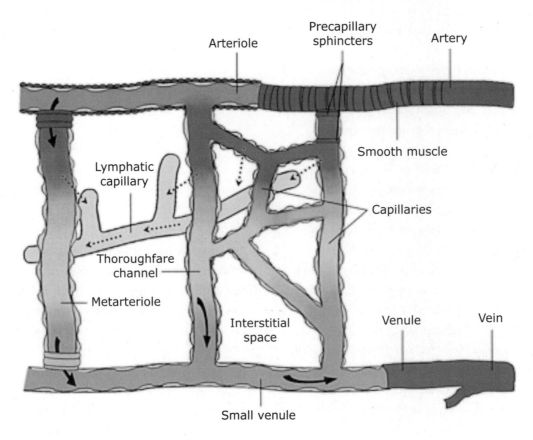

Figure 1.
Scioli et al. Aging and microvasculature. *Vascular Cell*. 2014;6:19.

20. The gas that diffuses out of the capillaries and into the interstitial fluid is
  a. CO_2
  b. NH_3
  c. O_2
  d. N_2

21. Based on the fluid movement described in the passage, the osmotic pressure on the arteriole end of the capillary bed is
  a. greater than the hydrostatic pressure.
  b. less than the hydrostatic pressure.
  c. equal to the hydrostatic pressure.
  d. bidirectional on the capillary walls.

22. If all arterial blood is directed into the capillary bed, the flow rate of the blood in the capillaries should
  a. increase, per Dalton's law.
  b. decrease, per Dalton's law.
  c. increase, per the continuity equation.
  d. decrease, per the continuity equation.

23. Which of the following assumptions of Poiseuille's equation is true of capillary bed blood flow and does not demonstrate the limitations of the equation in this context?
  a. The fluid is Newtonian.
  b. The fluid is incompressible.
  c. The tube is long and straight.
  d. Fluid flow is steady and laminar.

24. Heat transfer due to concerted, collective movement within fluids is

a. conductive.

b. convective.

c. mechanical.

d. radiative.

25. Pressure-volume (PV) diagrams are widely used to characterize the performance of the intact heart under various conditions. For a particular cavity of the heart, the point at the bottom right of the loop is the end-diastolic point where the contraction begins. Moving counterclockwise around the loop, the opening and closing of the cavity's valves react to changes in pressure and volume. The upper left curve of the loop represents the end-systolic point. The PV diagram below was recorded for simultaneous contractions of the left (outer, larger loop) and right (inner, smaller loop) ventricles of the heart.

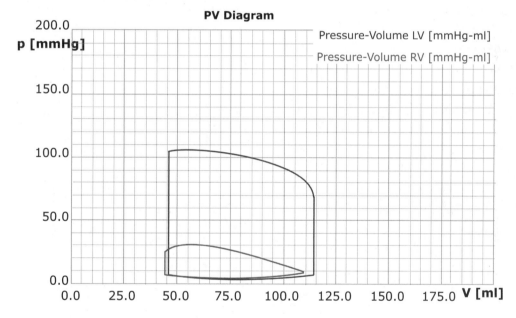

Wildhaber et al. A graphical simulation software for instruction in cardiovascular mechanics physiology. *BioMedical Engineering OnLine.* 2011;10:8.

What conclusion can be drawn about the behavior of the left and right ventricles under the tested conditions?

a. The end-systolic volume is higher than the end-diastolic volume for both the left and right ventricles during ventricular contraction.

b. The contraction of the left ventricle contributes more than that of the right ventricle to the total amount of work done by the ventricles to eject blood.

c. The elasticity of the right ventricle is significantly lower than normal under the conditions tested in the experiment, while the elasticity of the left ventricle has not been affected.

d. The elasticity of the left ventricle is significantly higher than normal under the conditions tested in the experiment, while the elasticity of the right ventricle has not been affected.

26. The change in length of an object under linear thermal expansion is a function of

      I. the initial length

      II. the initial temperature

      III. the magnitude of change in temperature

  a. I only

  b. I and II only

  c. I and III only

  d. I, II, and III

Questions 27 through 31 are based on the following passage.

Ribonuclease L (RNase L) is a key antiviral endoribonuclease that is induced and activated by virus infection, interferons, or double-stranded RNA (dsRNA). A cofactor called 2-5A binds to monomeric RNase L to convert it to an active, dimeric enzyme. When active, dimeric RNase L degrades single-stranded RNA to eliminate virus and virus-infected cells.

Curcumin, an orange-yellow pigment from the herb *c. longa*, has been found to have numerous therapeutic effects. The chemical structure is shown in Figure 1. Its effect on RNase L activity was studied. The interaction was determined to follow Michaelis-Menten kinetics.

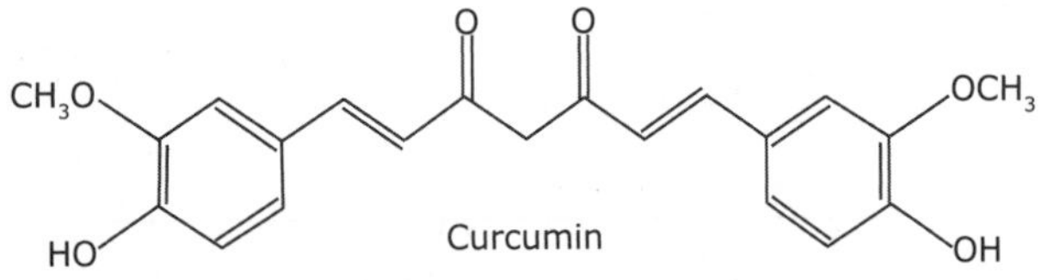

Figure 1. The chemical structure of curcumin.

Reaction mixtures were prepared that contained purified protein, 2-5A, and 0, 5, or 10 µM curcumin. RNA degradation was quantified by measuring the intensity of the residual intact bands of 28S and 18S rRNAs in each reaction and subtracting it from that of a background control reaction containing no 2-5A cofactor. Using this method, Michaelis-Menten curves were created to test the effect of curcumin on RNase L activity (Figure 2). With curcumin present, the K_m did not change, but V_{max} decreased.

Finally, the change in intrinsic fluorescence intensity $[(F_0-F)/F_0]$ from a 280-nm excitation wavelength at the 340-nm emission wavelength was measured with increasing curcumin concentrations in order to test the ability of the molecule to bind RNase L (Figure 3; page 57). The K_d value for binding was determined by fitting the curve using the Hill equation.

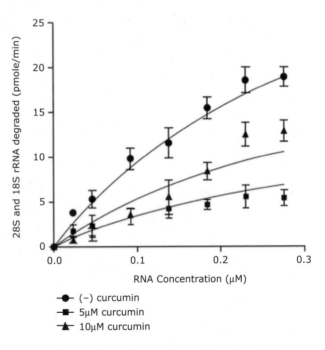

Figure 2. The effect of curcumin on RNase L activity.

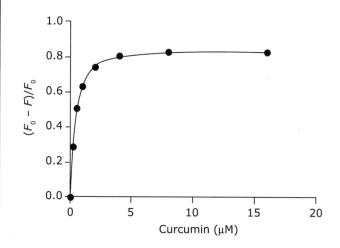

Figure 3. Fluorescence-based binding of curcumin to RNase L.

Source: Ankush Gupta and Pramod C. Rath, "Curcumin, a Natural *Antioxidant, Acts as a Noncompetitive Inhibitor of Human RNase L in Presence of Its Cofactor 2-5A in Vitro,*" *BioMed Research International*, vol. 2014, Article ID 817024, 9 pages, 2014. doi:10.1155/2014/817024.

27. Curcumin, shown in Figure 1, has a characteristic UV-visible spectral peak around 419 nm. The structural feature of curcumin that is most responsible for this UV-visible signal is its
a. anhydride group.
b. hydroxyl groups.
c. spin-spin splitting.
d. conjugated π-system.

28. Which Lineweaver-Burk plot most resembles the effect of curcumin (dashed line) on normal RNase L activity (solid line)?

a.
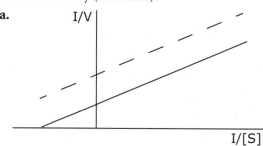

b.
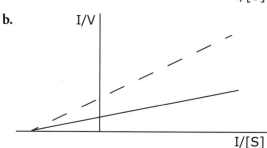

c.
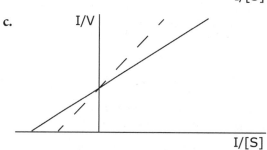

d. The line does not change when inhibitor is added.

29. Based on the data collected in these experiments, what is the mode of RNase L inhibition by curcumin?
a. Competitive inhibition
b. Uncompetitive inhibition
c. Noncompetitive inhibition
d. Irreversible inhibition

30. The most significant contributors to the intrinsic fluorescence and curcumin-induced quenching, measured in Figure 3, are

  a. tryptophan residues.
  b. alanine residues.
  c. cysteine residues.
  d. glutamine residues.

31. How can the Gibbs free energy of curcumin binding to RNase L be determined from the data obtained in these experiments?

  a. $\Delta G = RT \ln(K_d)$

  b. $\Delta G = \dfrac{V_{max}}{\text{[Total RNase L Concentration]}}$

  c. $\Delta G = K_d\left(1 + \dfrac{\text{[Curcumin Concentration]}}{K_i}\right)$

  d. $\Delta G = e^{K_d/RT}$

Questions 32 through 35 are based on the following passage.

The human eye is the organ that reacts to light. The outer layer of the eye is called the cornea. The cornea has a refractive index (n) of 1.38 and a radius of curvature (R) of 7.8 mm. Air has a refractive index of 1.00, while water has a refractive index of 1.33. The average distance from the cornea to the retina is 17.0 mm. Myopia, or nearsightedness, occurs when rays are focused before they reach the retina, while hyperopia, or farsightedness, occurs when light rays focus behind the retina rather than directly on it.

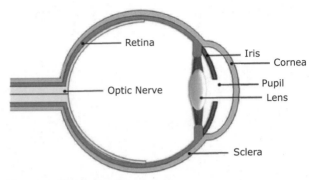

Figure 1. The human eye.
Samantha L. Wilson, Alicia J. El Haj, Ying Yang. Control of scar tissue formation in the cornea: Strategies in clinical and corneal tissue engineering. *J Funct Biomater.* 2012;3(3):642–687.

32. What percentage of its refracting power does the cornea lose when submerged in water compared to the open air?

  $\text{Refracting power} = \dfrac{n_1 - n_2}{d \text{ (in meters)}}$

  a. 13%
  b. 25%
  c. 75%
  d. 87%

33. What is the effective focal length, f, for the average eye for an object that is positioned 1.00 meter away in the open air?

  $\dfrac{1}{f} = \dfrac{1}{d_0} + \dfrac{1}{d_i}$

  a. 0.0598 mm
  b. 0.598 mm
  c. 1.67 mm
  d. 16.7 mm

34. A ray of light passes from the open air into the cornea at an incident angle of 80.0°. From Snell's Law, what is the angle of refraction in the cornea?

  a. 10.0°
  b. 44.5°
  c. 45.5°
  d. 80.0°

35. Based on Figure 1 (page 58) and the information in the passage, which of the following is a possible cause of myopia?
 a. There is insufficient optical (refractive) power.
 b. The eye is too long.
 c. The refractive index of the cornea constantly fluctuates.
 d. There are defects in the retinal ganglia.

36. Circular dichroism (CD) spectroscopy makes use of the differential absorption of left and right circularly polarized light to study the secondary structure of proteins. Circularly polarized light occurs when
 a. the oscillation of the electric field occurs in one plane.
 b. the electric field vector rotates in a plane perpendicular to the propagation direction with increasing angular velocity.
 c. the electric field vector rotates in a plane perpendicular to the propagation direction with constant angular velocity.
 d. the electric field vector rotates in a plane perpendicular to the propagation direction with decreasing angular velocity.

37. Saponification is the process of soap formation using a triglyceride as the starting molecule. The saponification reaction is
 a. the alkaline oxidation of aldehydes.
 b. the alkaline hydrolysis of esters.
 c. the acidic cleavage of glycols.
 d. acidic reduction of carboxylic acids.

38. The type of radioactive decay that does NOT change the atomic number of a nucleus is
 a. α decay.
 b. β decay.
 c. γ decay.
 d. electron capture.

Questions 39 through 44 are based on the following passage.

Arginase (RocF) hydrolyzes L-arginine to form L-ornithine and urea [$CO(NH_2)_2$]. In general, arginases have an alkaline pH optimum and require manganese for activation, but the *Helicobacter pylori* is optimally active with cobalt at pH 6. The metal ion forms a complex with arginine and promotes the enzymatic reaction. The arginase from *Bacillus anthracis* was purified for a structural and functional investigation.

The *B. anthracis rocF* gene was cloned and expressed in *E. coli*. After purification, RocF was tested for arginase activity with several different metals. Arginase activity of extracts containing the expressed protein was measured at pH 6.3 and pH 9 in the presence of a wide array of metals, each individually tested at 5 mM, or using deionized water in a "no metal" control. Spectrophotometric readings were taken at 515 nm after 24 hours (Figure 1; page 60). A viable cell arginase assay was performed by growing *B. anthracis* in the absence or presence of various metal concentrations, and cells were harvested and assayed directly for arginase activity at its optimal pH (Figure 2). Finally, amino acid sequence alignment studies showed particularly high sequence conservation in a –DAHGD-residue string at the putative metal binding site.

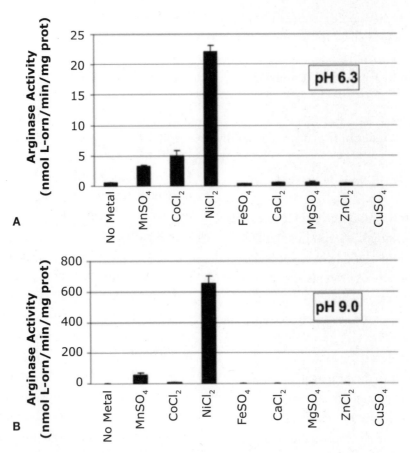

Figure 1. Arginase assay results for RocF activity in the presence of several different metals at pH 6.3 (A) and pH 9.0 (B).

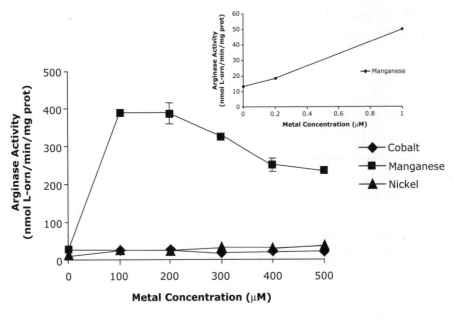

Figure 2. Viable cell arginase assay results in the presence of three metals of interest.
Ryan J. Viator, Richard F. Rest, Ellen Hildebrandt, David J. McGee. *BMC Biochemistry*. 2008;9:15. doi:10.1186/1471-2091-9-15.
These images are available from http://www.biomedcentral.com/1471-2091/9/15. © 2008 Viator et al; licensee BioMed Central Ltd.

39. Which of the tested metal ions has the largest ionic radius?

a. Mg^{2+}

b. Ca^{2+}

c. Ni^{2+}

d. Zn^{2+}

40. Based on the description of the arginase reaction in the passage, what is the structure of L-ornithine?

a.

b.

c.

d.

41. In comparison with arginase from *H. pylori*, RocF from *b. anthracis* has

a. the same metal preference and optimal pH.

b. the same metal preference but a different optimal pH.

c. a different metal preference but the same optimal pH.

d. a different metal preference and a different optimal pH.

42. The data in Figure 1 (page 60) directly show that changing the pH from 6.3 to 9 effectively changes

a. the binding affinity of RocF for each metal.

b. the ability of *b. anthracis* cells to survive in the presence of each metal.

c. the overall order of metal preference in RocF.

d. the rate of the arginase reaction in RocF for each metal.

43. The table below provides the pK_a values for several relevant amino acids in the structure of RocF:

AMINO ACID NAME	1-LETTER AMINO ACID CODE	SIDE CHAIN pK_a
Alanine	A	Not ionizable
Aspartate	D	3.9
Glycine	G	Not ionizable
Histidine	H	6.0

Assuming that pK_as are not affected by the surrounding protein structure, the majority (at least three) of the five residues in the conserved putative metal binding site are

a. uncharged at pH 6.3 and 9.0.

b. charged at pH 6.3 and 9.0.

c. aromatic.

d. hydrophobic.

44. The data collected in Figures 1 and 2
collectively suggest that, in vivo, *b. anthracis*

    a. cannot grow in the presence of Co^{2+} and
Ni^{2+}, even though RocF preferentially uses
these metals.

    b. specifically and efficiently imports Mn^{2+}, but
not Co^{2+} or Ni^{2+}, preventing RocF from
using its preferred metal.

    c. does not exhibit arginase activity at all
unless the protein is expressed and purified
in *E. coli*.

    d. exhibits the most rapid rate of arginase
activity at very low Mn^{2+} concentrations.

Questions 45 through 49 are based on the following passage.

The Prins reaction is the acid-catalyzed addition of aldehydes to alkenes. A general scheme for the Prins reaction is shown in Figure 1. With water and a protic acid as the reaction medium, the 1,3-diol is the reaction product. When water is absent, the allylic alcohol forms. A molar excess of formaldehyde and reaction temperature lower than 70°C gives the dioxane product. The replacement of water with acetic acid forms the corresponding esters.

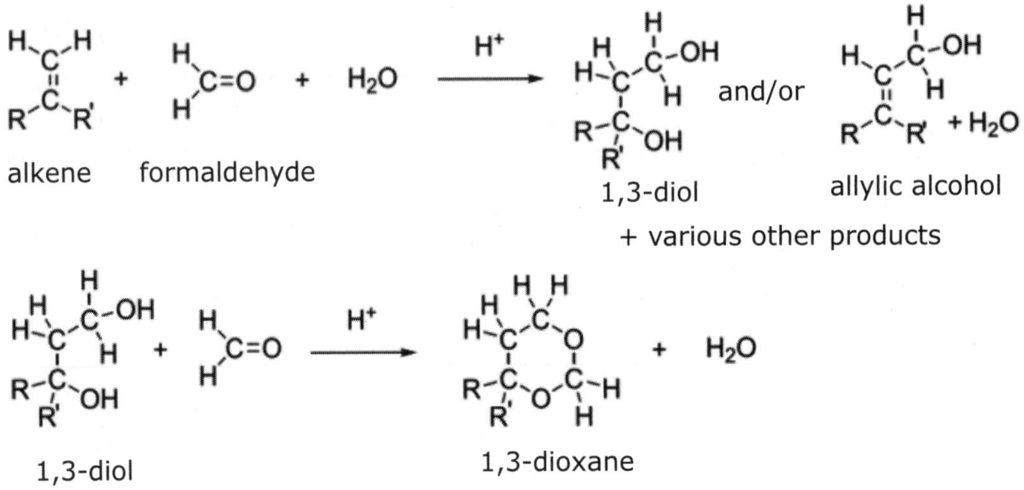

Figure 1. A general scheme for the Prins reaction.

    In a putative general mechanism for the Prins reaction using formaldehyde, the first step is the protonation of the oxygen in formaldehyde to form a carbocation, followed by the addition of the alkene ($CH_2 =$ CRR') to form a new carbocation X (Figure 2A). Carbocation X then reacts with water to form the 1,3-diol. The 1,3-diol is then protonated at its alcohol, forming water as a leaving group, which makes the allylic alcohol product. Carbocation X also reacts with the aldehyde to form a linear ether–containing carbocation, which cyclizes to form the 1,3-dioxane product.

The Prins reaction was performed by reacting isobutylene (Figure 2B) with formaldehyde. The main products formed are 75% 1,3-dioxane (Figure 2C) and 9% 1,3-diol.

A   **B**   **C**

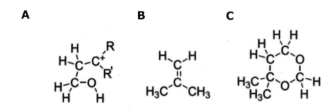

Figure 2. Relevant intermediates, reactants, and products for the Prins reaction. A, carbocation X; B, isobutylene; C, 1,3-dioxane.

Shinichi Yamabe, Takeshi Fukuda, Shoko Yamazaki. Beilstein *J Org Chem*, 2013, 9, 476–485. This passage contains excerpts from this work. The entire article can be found at http://www.beilstein-journals.org/bjoc/content/pdf/1860-5397-9-51.pdf.

45. In the general Prins reaction mechanism, why does the CH_2 carbon of the alkene, and not the CRR' carbon, bond with the carbon on the protonated formaldehyde to form X (Figure 2)?

    a. The electronegativity difference between C and H in the C-H bonds of the alkene gives the CH_2 carbon slightly less electron pull than the CRR' carbon.

    b. The bond formation with the CH_2 carbon over the CRR' carbon forms a more stable tertiary carbocation.

    c. Mechanistically, this mode of bond formation provides the most stable pi bond arrangement, according to Hückel's rule.

    d. The bond formation with the CH_2 carbon over the CRR' carbon is less sterically favorable, but the bond energy of the new bond is significantly higher.

46. The formation of the allylic alcohol from 1,3-diol is

    a. an elimination reaction.

    b. a hydrolysis reaction.

    c. a tautomerization reaction.

    d. a nucleophilic substitution reaction.

47. Which set of reaction conditions could have been used to obtain the products in the isobutylene Prins reaction with formaldehyde described in the passage?

    a. $(CH_3)_2CO$ (aq), 32°C, 3:4 alkene:formaldehyde molar ratio

    b. H_2SO_4 (aq), 32°C, 3:4 alkene:formaldehyde molar ratio

    c. $(CH_3)_2CO$ (aq), 75°C, 4:3 alkene:formaldehyde molar ratio

    d. H_2SO_4 (aq), 75°C, 4:3 alkene:formaldehyde molar ratio

48. What is the correct IUPAC name of the 1,3-diol that forms during the isobutylene Prins reaction with formaldehyde?

    a. 1,1-dimethyl-1,3-propanediol

    b. 2,2-dimethyl-1,2-propanediol

    c. 2-methyl-2,4-butanediol

    d. 3-methyl-1,3-butanediol

49. What is the orbital hybridization of the oxygen atoms in 1,3-dioxane?

    a. sp

    b. sp^2

    c. sp^3

    d. sp^3d

Questions 50 through 52 are based on the following passage.

Lysergic acid diethylamide (LSD) is a psychedelic drug and powerful hallucinogen that was first synthesized in 1938 from ergotamine, a chemical derived from a grain fungus that often grows on rye. The chemical structure of LSD is shown in Figure 1, with its three nitrogen atoms numbered 1–3 and with carbon 8 labeled C-8.

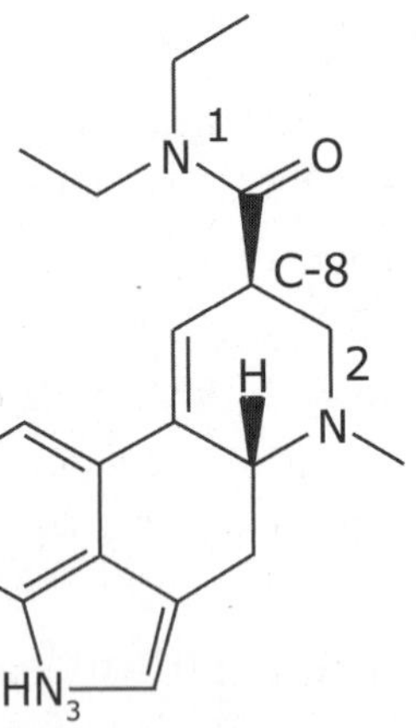

Figure 1. The chemical structure of lysergic acid diethylamide.

50. How many unique stereoisomers are possible for the LSD molecule?
   a. 1
   b. 2
   c. 4
   d. 8

51. Based on the structure of LSD, which of the nitrogen atoms in the molecule is the most basic?
   a. Nitrogen atom 1
   b. Nitrogen atom 2
   c. Nitrogen atom 3
   d. All three nitrogen atoms are equally basic.

52. Why is the proton on C-8 labile?
   a. The carboxamide group on the molecule is electron withdrawing.
   b. The pi electron delocalization on the indole ring and the nearby nitrogen are electron withdrawing.
   c. The steric stress from bulky groups increases the lability of the C-8 proton.
   d. The structural stress from the planarity of LSD increases the lability of the C-8 proton.

53. The stretching frequencies of several functional groups are shown below:

FUNCTIONAL GROUPS	STRETCHING FREQUENCIES (WAVENUMBERS)
Alcohols	3590–3650
Alkanes	2800–3000
Alkenes	3000–3100
Amines	3300–3500 (doublet for NH_2)
Aromatics	1500–1600
Carboxylic Acids	2500–3300
Nitriles	2220–2260

Using the table of functional groups, which molecule corresponds with the infrared (IR) spectrum below?

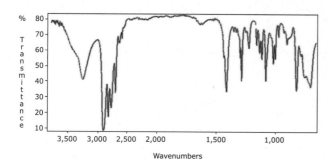

a.

b. H_3C——N

c.

d.

54. Sulfur dioxide reacts with oxygen in an enclosed container as follows:

$$2SO_2(g) + O_2(g) \rightleftharpoons 2SO_3(g) \ \Delta H = -198.2 \ kJ$$

Which of the following changes will shift the equilibrium to the left?
a. Adding a catalyst
b. Adding O_2
c. Decreasing the pressure
d. Decreasing the temperature

55. Plant sucrose uptake transporters (SUTs) are H^+/sucrose symporters, and OsSUT1 is a type II SUT. The OsSUT1(R188K) mutant was made that replaced lysine with arginine at position 188, altering a key residue in the transmembrane portion of the protein. R188H and R188M mutants did not localize to the membrane. ^{14}C sucrose uptake by yeast expressing wildtype OsSUT1, the mutant, and an empty pDR196 gene vector was measured at pH 4.0 and 7.0, at 30°C for 5 minutes each. The results are shown in the graph below:

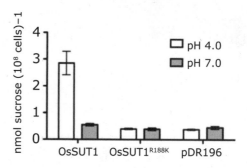

Sun and Ward. Arg188 in rice sucrose transporter OsSUT1 is crucial for substrate transport. *BMC Biochemistry.* 2012;13:26.

Based on the results obtained, OsSUT1 will localize and function properly at pH 4.0 as long as residue 188
a. is positively charged.
b. can form a bidentate H-bond.
c. is hydrophobic.
d. has a low enough molecular weight.

56. Consider the following redox reaction acidic solution:

$$H_2S + NO_3^- \rightarrow S_8 + NO$$

When balanced using the smallest possible integers, the coefficient for H_2S is

a. 4.

b. 8.

c. 16.

d. 24.

57. The following data were obtained for this hypothetical reaction:

$$A + B \rightarrow C$$

$[A]_0$, mM	$[B]_0$, mM	INITIAL RATE OF [C] PRODUCTION (mM/s)
120	170	4,705
360	170	4,698
360	340	18,800

Based on the data, which of the following measurements should be linear, with slope k or $-k$, as a function of time?

a. $[A]$

b. $[B]$

c. $[A]^{-1}$

d. $[B]^{-1}$

58. Fractional distillation is a method used to separate two or more liquids in the same mixture. This method relies on differences between the liquids in

a. polarity.

b. density.

c. boiling point.

d. solubility in two distinct solvents.

59. The Lewis acid-base reaction between boron trifluoride and ethanol produces

a. one zwitterionic compound.

b. one charged compound.

c. two neutral compounds.

d. two charged compounds.

$$CH_3OH + BF_3 \rightleftharpoons CH_3 - \overset{\overset{\displaystyle H}{|}}{\underset{\oplus}{O}} - \overset{\ominus}{BF_3}$$

Part 3: Psychological, Social, and Biological Foundations of Behavior

59 Questions
95 Minutes

Use the following passage to answer questions 1 through 5.

An experimenter wanted to see if a new form of teaching would help accelerate the cognitive development of eighth- and ninth-grade science students. He hypothesized that the new method, a "flipped" classroom method where students worked on homework and group assignments in class and listened to lectures at home, would accelerate the students' cognitive development. To test this hypothesis, students were randomly assigned into two groups. One group was taught a concept in the traditional lecture method in class, while the other was given the "flipped" classroom method. After eight weeks, the experimenter compared scores of both groups using the same critical thinking assessment. The results suggested that although there was a great deal of variability within each group and cognitive development did improve in some students, overall there were no statistically significant differences between the traditional lecture and the "flipped" classroom conditions.

1. Based on the information in the passage, whose developmental theory was this study grounded in?
   a. Erikson's
   b. Freud's
   c. Maslow's
   d. Piaget's

2. According the theories upon which this study is based, children in the concrete operational stage have problems with which of the following?
   a. Deductive logic
   b. Perspective taking
   c. Inductive logic
   d. Conservation

3. If the treatment in this study were considered to be a stressor, what was the effect of the stressor on the children who succeeded in the study?
   a. They did best if they received the familiar to unfamiliar treatment.
   b. They moved from one developmental stage to the next.
   c. They were relaxed, so they did well in the study.
   d. They were better at combinatorial reasoning than propositional logic.

4. The study compared the group means on a critical thinking assessment. What type of statistics are used when comparing the means of groups?
   a. Inferential
   b. Estimation
   c. Descriptive
   d. Modeling

5. What physiological change occurs in children as they move from concrete operational to formal operational stages of cognitive development?
   a. The limbic system is altered.
   b. Changes in the brain occur in the memory storage area.
   c. Psychological functioning changes, but the structure of the brain does not change.
   d. The structure of the brain changes.

6. Which of the following is a correlation that BEST supports Maslow's hierarchy of needs?

a. Children living in poverty tend to be victims of violent crime.

b. Children living in poverty and/or in violent neighborhoods tend to do less well in school than their affluent peers.

c. Children who interact with their environment develop deeper knowledge structures than children who do not.

d. Children who receive scaffolded instruction learn relationships between concepts faster than those who do not.

7. The sense of having always known a person whom we just met is an example of which of the following in romantic love?

a. Attachment

b. Attraction

c. Love

d. Lust

8. Which part of the brain confers an evolutionary advantage by allowing parallel processing?

a. Only the right brain

b. Only the left brain

c. Conus medullaris

d. Lateralization of cortical functions

9. Spatial cognition and cognitive mapping are often found in which of the following?

a. Reinforcement schedules

b. Avoidance learning

c. Spontaneous recovery

d. Associative learning

Use the following passage to answer questions 10 through 14.

Social thinking is what we do when we interact with people: we think about them. And how we think about people affects how we behave, which in turn affects how others respond to us, which in turn affects our own emotions. Whether we are with friends, sending an e-mail, in a classroom, or at the grocery store, we take in the thoughts, emotions, and intentions of the people we are interacting with.

Most of us develop our communications sense from birth onward, steadily observing and acquiring social information and learning how to respond to people. Because social thinking is an intuitive process, we usually take it for granted.

But for many individuals, this process is anything but natural. And this often has nothing to do with conventional measures of intelligence. In fact, many people score high on IQ and standardized tests yet do not intuitively learn the nuances of social communication and interaction.

While these challenges are commonly experienced by individuals with autism spectrum disorders (high functioning), social communication disorder, Asperger's, attention deficit hyperactivity disorder (ADHD), nonverbal learning disability (NLD), and similar diagnoses, children and adults experiencing social learning difficulties often have received no diagnosis.

A treatment framework and curriculum developed by Michelle Garcia Winner targets improving individual social thinking abilities, regardless of diagnostic label. Professionals and parents alike are using these methods to build social thinking and related skills in students and adults. Social thinking books, workshops, and trainings by Winner or based on Winner's work now offer a range of strategies that address individual strengths and weaknesses in processing social information.

Research is beginning to support the effectiveness of teaching social thinking. The *Journal of Autism and Developmental Disorders* published a report on methodologies specifically addressing weaknesses in the social thinking process, finding that they are successful at teaching the ability to interact socially in people with social limitations who have near-average to very high intelligence.

10. Based on the article, which of the following is TRUE?
   a. All people experiencing social thinking difficulties have a diagnosis.
   b. Parents are using strategies to help their children overcome social thinking difficulties.
   c. Research does not support teaching methodologies that claim to help overcome social thinking difficulties.
   d. Most social learning occurs during preadolescence and adolescence.

11. Interventions have been developed for people with social thinking difficulties. Which of the following is MOST correct about these interventions?
   a. Social thinking is a natural process for everyone, so interventions have not been effective.
   b. Only people best at social thinking have high IQs, so interventions have focused on individuals with lower IQs.
   c. Interventions on social thinking have found that the interventions are effective with people who have high IQs.
   d. There are few interventions available, and those are directed at individuals with diagnostic labels.

12. If a type of social thinking intervention were to be tested using experimental design, the outcome of the experiment would be MOST related to which of the following?
   a. Control group
   b. Dependent variable
   c. Experimental group
   d. Independent variable

13. Why do most people take social thinking for granted?
   a. It is closely related to IQ, which means it is an intuitive process.
   b. It is learned quickly from the environment, so most people do not even notice it.
   c. Most people who have trouble with social thinking have a diagnosis, so for those without a diagnosis, it is an intuitive process.
   d. It is an intuitive process, so it is not noticed, even in the most severe cases.

14. What is unique about Winner's work on social thinking?
   a. It is being used not only by practitioners but also by parents.
   b. It can only be used with patients with a secondary diagnosis.
   c. It is not based on research on social thinking and has not contributed to the field.
   d. It has failed to help people with near-average to above-average intelligence.

Use the following passage to answer questions 15 through 19.

The term *mental illness* clearly indicates that there is a problem with the mind. But is it just the mind in an abstract sense, or is there a physical basis to mental illness? As scientists continue to investigate mental illnesses and their causes, they learn more and more about how the biological processes that make the brain work are changed when a person has a mental illness.

How does the brain take in all of this information, process it, and cause a response? The basic functional unit of the brain is the neuron. A neuron is a specialized cell that can produce different actions because of its precise connections with other neurons, sensory receptors, and muscle cells. A typical neuron has four structurally and functionally defined regions: the cell body, dendrites, axons, and axon terminals.

When the electrical signal reaches the presynaptic axon terminal, it cannot cross the synaptic space, or synaptic cleft. Instead, the electrical signal triggers chemical changes that *can* cross the synapse to affect the postsynaptic cell. When the electrical impulse reaches the presynaptic axon terminal, membranous sacs called vesicles move toward the membrane of the axon terminal. When the vesicles reach the membrane, they fuse with the membrane and release their contents into the synaptic space. The molecules contained in the vesicles are chemical compounds called neurotransmitters.

The nervous system uses a variety of neurotransmitter molecules, but each neuron specializes in the synthesis and secretion of a single type of neurotransmitter. Some of the predominant neurotransmitters in the brain include glutamate, GABA, serotonin, dopamine, and norepinephrine. Each of these neurotransmitters has a specific distribution and function in the brain.

Research scientists want to learn about the chemical or structural changes that occur in the brain when someone has a mental illness. If scientists can determine what happens in the brain, they can use that knowledge to develop better treatments or find a cure. At this time, scientists do not have a complete understanding of what causes mental illnesses. If you think about the structural and organizational complexity of the brain, together with the complex effects that mental illnesses have on thoughts, feelings, and behaviors, it is hardly surprising that figuring out the causes of mental illnesses is a daunting task.

Most scientists believe that mental illnesses result from problems with the communication between neurons in the brain. For example, the level of the neurotransmitter serotonin is lower in individuals who have depression. This finding led to the development of certain medications for the illness. Selective serotonin reuptake inhibitors (SSRIs) work by reducing the amount of serotonin that is taken back into the presynaptic neuron. This leads to an increase in the amount of serotonin available in the synaptic space for binding to the receptor on the postsynaptic neuron. Changes in other neurotransmitters (in addition to serotonin) may occur in depression, thus adding to the complexity of the cause underlying the disease.

Scientists believe that there may be disruptions in the neurotransmitters dopamine, glutamate, and norepinephrine in individuals who have schizophrenia. One indication that dopamine might be an important neurotransmitter in schizophrenia comes from the observation that cocaine addicts sometimes show symptoms similar to schizophrenia. Cocaine acts on dopamine-containing neurons in the brain to increase the amount of dopamine in the synapse.

15. Where in the structure of the neuron are neurotransmitters found?
  a. At the axon of the presynaptic neuron
  b. In vesicles located at the presynaptic axon terminal
  c. In the dendrite
  d. In the cytoplasmic connection between the two neurons

16. Schizophrenia is likely to be caused in cocaine users by an increase of which of the following neurotransmitters?
  a. Serotonin
  b. Glutamate
  c. Dopamine
  d. Norepinephrine

17. Which of the following are MOST likely to experience vicarious emotional trauma when dealing with mental illness?
  a. Mental health workers
  b. Patients with bipolar disorder
  c. Patients with alcoholism
  d. Patients with schizophrenia

18. Dysfunctional mirror neuro activity (MNA) may be found in which of the following mental conditions?
  a. Bipolar disorder and major depression
  b. PTSD and eating disorders
  c. Obsessive-compulsive disorder and antisocial personality disorder
  d. Autism and schizophrenia

19. Mental disorders such as generalized anxiety disorder are generally caused by problems with which of the following?
  a. Axons
  b. Neurons
  c. Neurotransmitters
  d. Substance abuse

Use the following passage to answer questions 20 through 24.

A North American middle school was the setting of a research study about the implementation of an intervention to prevent gendered harassment. The teachers in the school ($n = 70$) were divided into two groups ($n = 35$ each), one that received the intervention and one that did not. All of the teachers in the school participated in the study. The intervention included a week-long training during the summer about gender roles, gender identification, and gendered harassment. A major component of the training was to have the teachers identify and confront their limiting beliefs about gender identity in general and gender in preadolescents in particular. This process upset many of the teachers to the point where six teachers almost dropped out of the study. However, all six worked through their feelings and made the commitment to continue in the study. During the fall semester of the school year, the teachers in the intervention group met a minimum of twice a week for 30 minutes to discuss in small groups the issues they were facing, and specific challenges were addressed. The researchers also met with the participants in a large group once a month for a 2-hour debriefing to discuss issues raised by the small groups and to provide additional training as necessary. Teachers in the intervention group also were encouraged to keep a diary, personal blog, or some other record of their experiences. All 35 began the diary process, but only 27 used it consistently during the intervention. Some of these teachers went even further and formed online groups. The entire school-based portion of the intervention lasted one semester (15 weeks).

Data were collected in the following manner from all 70 teachers and their students. Classroom observations were made during weeks 1 and 2, weeks 7 and 8, and weeks 14 and 15. All teachers were interviewed at the beginning and end of the study.

Students were given a Likert-type questionnaire during weeks 1 and 15. This questionnaire was administered in a single setting. There was one significant difference on the student questionnaire at the beginning of the study, which was that transgender students were more likely to report feeling bullied. Qualitative data were quantified where appropriate, and statistical tests of significance were performed. The observational data showed that the teachers who were in the intervention group were more effective at dealing with incidents of bullying at the times they occurred than the nonintervention group. The students of the teachers in the intervention group were significantly less likely to express or conversely be the victims of gendered harassment after the intervention. For the nonintervention group, perceived lack of administrative support and lack of training were the most common reasons given for failure to deal with gendered harassment in the classroom. Both groups expressed fear of parental backlash and lack of community conformity as reasons that gendered harassment interventions may not be very effective.

20. The teachers who did NOT receive the intervention in the study are referred to as which of the following?
    a. Control group
    b. Experimental group
    c. Dependent variable
    d. Independent variable

21. Based on the results of the study, which of the following is a reasonable conclusion that can be made about gendered harassment interventions?
    a. The programs work if teachers and administrators are committed to them.
    b. The programs were proven effective at reducing bullying in the classroom.
    c. Putting bullying students through similar interventions will reduce their tendency to bully.
    d. Community conformity is a contributing factor that can lead to the lack of success of these programs.

22. During the teacher learning phase, several teachers had personal experiences that led to a decision to almost drop out of the program. All eventually stayed. Which is the best term for these teachers' personal experiences?
    a. Adaptation
    b. Cognitive dissonance
    c. Cultural conformity
    d. Independent variable

23. Which variable in this study is socially constructed?
    a. Gender
    b. Sex
    c. Age of students
    d. Treatment length

24. Which of the following statements is an example of a view consistent with the hidden curriculum in the context of this study?

   a. Students with different gender identities get bullied because it prepares them for real-life discrimination.

   b. The nature of the bullying intervention was known only to the teachers and not to the students.

   c. Bullying is unacceptable in all situations.

   d. Bullying is the fault of parents.

25. A family immigrates to a new country and strives to fit in. The parents insist the children speak only the new language in the home, and the adults strive to join many social groups and make many new friends from their new country. Which term is this cultural process is known as?

   a. Accommodation

   b. Assimilation

   c. Functionalism

   d. Stratification

26. All of the following are forms of signals that animals use, EXCEPT

   a. adaptation.

   b. gaze following.

   c. electrocommunication.

   d. olfactory.

27. Which of the following was the first theory of motivation?

   a. Incentive theory

   b. Arousal theory

   c. Humanistic theory

   d. Drive reduction theory

Use the following chart to answer questions 28 through 32.

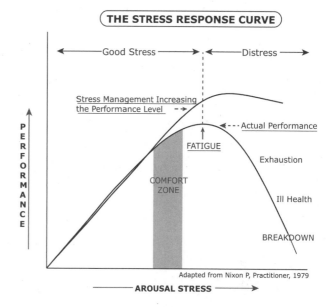

Adapted from Nixon P, Practitioner, 1979

28. According to the graph, at what point is stress no longer beneficial?

   a. When side effects to health occur

   b. When the comfort zone is achieved

   c. When performance is maximized

   d. When fatigue occurs

29. If an experiment were performed to compare the difference between one group receiving stress management treatment and the other group not receiving treatment, what kind of research design would be used?

   a. Case study

   b. Experimental

   c. Cross-sectional

   d. Descriptive

30. The information in the graph is based on the work of which of the following theorists?
  a. Cannon-Bard
  b. James-Lange
  c. Piaget-Maslow
  d. Schachter-Singer

31. An experiment was performed to compare the difference between one group receiving stress management treatment and the other group not receiving treatment. A requirement of the study was to turn in a signed IRB form. Subject X did not turn in his form by the time the study started but was considered by the research team to be a desirable subject for the study. What should the researchers do?
  a. Let Subject X participate without the form.
  b. Give Subject X a deadline of 2 weeks to turn in the form.
  c. Allow Subject X to be included as long as the form is turned in by the end of the study.
  d. Not allow Subject X to participate in the study because he did not follow study protocol.

32. While the theoretical constructs of the theory this graph was based on are now mostly obsolete, the relationship shown in the graph is an example of modern use. What is another example?
  a. A person is aroused and has no immediate explanation, so he labels this state and describes his feelings in terms of the thoughts available to him at the time.
  b. Crying and trembling in public, which is caused by the person's emotions.
  c. Becoming ill in public, which leads to anxiety, which leads to avoidance of being in public.
  d. Being anxious in public, which leads to avoidance of being in public.

Use the following passage to answer questions 33 through 37.

The New York Times notes that "more than 6 percent of American teenagers are clinically depressed." There are many different causes of teen depression, a disorder that can be a precursor to teen suicide attempts. Screening for teen depression is crucial and is now performed at the offices of many pediatricians. About 70 percent of teens with depression fail to seek medical treatment or therapy. Thus, parents must be proactive to watch for signs of depression in teens.

Daily life for teenagers is often stressful and causes many teenagers to feel tormented, isolated, and different from others. This stress may be a factor leading to depression. Problems such as bullying, violence, and gossip are part of daily life for teens. Since teens' brains are not yet fully developed, they do not have the logic skills to work through the difficult situations these experiences may create.

Teenagers who have to handle a lot of change in their lives may be more susceptible to bouts of depression. Major life changes such as the divorce of parents, loss of a friend or relationship, death in the family, unemployment of a parent, relocation away from friends, or sudden disability can cause enormous stress for a teenager. Teenagers may overreact to stress and changes in life and may succumb to negative thinking and depression.

If a teenager abuses alcohol or drugs, this may lead to depression. Alcohol is a depressant. Drug use may impair the brain's ability to function properly and impact the hormonal system, which can lead to depression. When depression arises, teens may limit social interaction, let grades drop, attempt suicide, drop out of school, stop participating in school activities, or fight with peers and parents. Teens under stress and using drugs and alcohol are susceptible to negative thinking, which can lead to depression.

As hormones surge in teenagers, they may feel overwhelmed by the changes in their bodies and their moods. They may experience foul moods, may have a hostile attitude, and may be involved in self-destructive acts such as cutting or promiscuous behavior. A teenager often does not understand the mood swings that surging hormones can create. They may become withdrawn and start to experience depression due to feeling out of control of their changing bodies.

Teenagers must work to avoid causes of depression and focus on the positive aspects of life. Ongoing exercise at least three times a week helps prevent depression. It is also helpful to spend time with positive and achievement-oriented friends. Participating in hobbies that bring joy is also helpful to prevent the onset of depression. Other ways to work to prevent depression include getting at least eight hours of sleep a night, avoiding pessimistic thoughts, talking to a doctor or guidance counselor if stressed or in crisis, eating healthy foods and avoiding junk food, avoiding sad music, and avoiding friends who abuse drugs or alcohol.

33. According to the article, which of the following is a stressor that can cause teens to be depressed?
    a. Peer pressure
    b. Daily exercise
    c. Cutting and promiscuity
    d. Reducing participation in school activities

34. Which agent of socialization is MOST likely to be the location of the stressors that cause depression?
    a. Mass media
    b. School
    c. Church
    d. Workplace

35. In what way does mass media influence teens' development?
    a. Teens tend to be very devoted to the music they listen to, and this influences their identity formation.
    b. Most teens tend to emulate the movie and television stars they admire, and this can influence their gender identity.
    c. Media usually positively affects their self-efficacy.
    d. Media influences their class identity.

36. Which social support system is MOST likely to help prevent teen depression?
    a. Church and church-related activities
    b. Friends in physical education class
    c. School
    d. Family

37. Low self-efficacy can MOST likely result from exposure to which of the following stressors?
    a. Family life
    b. Music, especially the music they listen to most
    c. Mass media, such as billboards and magazines
    d. Workplace

38. A child knows that thunder is caused by lightning but does not understand the causal mechanism between the two. In which stage of Piaget's developmental model does the child most likely belong?

    a. Concrete operational

    b. Formal operational

    c. Preoperational

    d. Sensory-motor

39. Which of the following is TRUE about ethnocentrism AND cultural relativism?

    a. They are only found in individuals.

    b. They are only found in specific nations.

    c. They are found in BOTH individuals and specific nations.

    d. They are found in NEITHER individuals nor specific nations.

40. Which of the following BEST describes groups making decisions that are more than the initial inclinations of its members?

    a. Deindividuation

    b. Deviance

    c. Groupthink

    d. Group polarization

41. Which of the following models or theories includes persuasion as a major component?

    a. Elaboration likelihood model

    b. Social cognitive theory

    c. Enculturation theory

    d. Observational learning model

42. A person going to an interview presents herself in a certain way, including speech, body language, and clothing. By doing so, she is practicing which of the following?

    a. Using gender in the detection of emotion

    b. Nonverbal communication

    c. Social interactionism

    d. Impression management

Use the following passage to answer questions 43 through 47.

Over the past few years, America's city centers have experienced revitalization. This has brought new life to cities and also put a premium on urban neighborhoods. Housing in such areas is scarce and often cannot grow at the rate that the population does. As an alternative, people are moving to and building homes in areas that were once considered undesirable. Gentrification often occurs in these areas, which have specific qualities that make them ideal. The biggest draw to these areas may be the availability of inexpensive housing, especially to younger generations who see older houses that haven't been maintained as "fixer-uppers" and investment opportunities.

Gentrification occurs through gradual increase in new people to a formerly undesirable neighborhood. At first, many people are unwilling or afraid to move into an unfamiliar neighborhood across class and racial lines. However, a small number of people do, and then through word of mouth, more people are willing to move. This snowball effect leads to an accelerated growth in an area that was once stagnating.

While gentrification has benefits, it also has consequences. As more people move to the new neighborhood, housing prices can become more and more inflated, as can the prices of food, gas, and other costs of living. In addition, although gentrification may bring vitality and economy to a neighborhood that once lacked these attributes, it often displaces the existing residents.

Despite this, gentrification supporters focus on the advantages of urban and environmental sustainability of city living. Policymakers are urging populations to live in highly populated cities contained within a small radius, in which mobility practices will become more localized. Although gentrification is being promoted as a way to sustain urban areas in the future, its success may leave those native to their existing communities without one.

43. Gentrification is most different from which of the following processes?
a. Meritocracy
b. Urban blight
c. Intergenerational mobility
d. Social stratification

44. A problem that people moving into gentrifying neighborhoods experience is MOST likely which of the following?
a. Healthcare disparities
b. Declining housing values
c. Global inequalities
d. Relative and absolute poverty

45. Which of the following will likely have to be improved because of gentrification?
a. The number of parks in the gentrified neighborhood
b. The variety of restaurants in the neighborhood
c. Availability of public transportation
d. The pace of change in the neighborhood

46. The children from the original neighborhood and children coming into the gentrified neighborhood may both experience all of the following within the education system EXCEPT
a. hidden curriculum.
b. in-group bias.
c. meritocracy.
d. displacement.

47. Which is most likely to occur in gentrified neighborhoods?
a. Assimilation of new families into existing culture
b. Poor families being driven out of their existing neighborhood
c. Less violence in the family
d. Culture lag

Use the following passage to answer questions 48 through 50.

A study was undertaken to determine if there were differences in the health beliefs, health locus of control, and self-concept of adult women who practice breast self-examination (BSE) compared with women who do not. A sample of 207 women, drawn from a variety of settings, completed four research instruments. Analysis of the data revealed differences between the practice and non-practice groups in terms of health beliefs, health locus of control, and self-concept, as well as a positive relationship between the measure of health belief and the measure of self-concept. Specifically, the group that practiced BSEs had higher levels of health beliefs and higher self-concept levels than the group that did not. Also, those who practiced BSEs tended to be less inclined to have a health locus of control that depended on a powerful other, in this case a physician.

48. In this study, the relationship between higher health beliefs and self-concept would be considered which of the following?
a. Correlational
b. Causal
c. Predictive
d. Variable

49. What is a locus of control?
   a. A psychological model that attempts to explain and predict behaviors related to issues like health
   b. An idea of the self, constructed from the beliefs one holds about oneself and the responses of others
   c. The extent to which individuals can control events affecting them
   d. One's confidence in one's own worth or abilities and one's self-respect

50. If an experiment was designed to train those in the non-practice group to start practicing BSEs, what would be the dependent variable in the study?
   a. The control group
   b. The treatment group
   c. The training the experimental group received
   d. Whether the group receiving the treatment started practicing breast self-exam

51. An on-duty nurse receives a call at the hospital in which the caller identifies himself as a doctor. He advises the nurse to give a large dose of medication to a patient. The highest allowable dose of the medication is 10 mg; however, the doctor advises the nurse to administer 20 mg. Despite the possible deadly consequences of such a high dose, the nurse administers the medication without asking any questions. This is an example of
   a. peer pressure.
   b. obedience.
   c. bystander effect.
   d. social loafing.

Use the following passage to answer questions 52 through 56.

A doctor is examining a CT scan, looking for evidence of a tumor. Either there is a tumor (signal present) or there is not (signal absent). Either the doctor sees a tumor (she responds "yes") or does not (she responds "no"). There are four possible outcomes: hit (tumor present and doctor says "yes"), miss (tumor present and doctor says "no"), false alarm (tumor absent and doctor says "yes"), or correct rejection (tumor absent and doctor says "no"). Hits and correct rejections are good. False alarms and misses are bad.

Detecting a tumor is difficult, and there will always be some amount of uncertainty. There are two kinds of noise factors that contribute to the uncertainty: *internal noise* and *external noise.*

External noise: There are many possible sources of external noise. There can be noise factors that are part of the photographic process, a smudge, or a bad spot on the film. Or there can be something in the person's lung that is fine but looks a bit like a tumor. All of these are examples of *external noise.*

Internal noise: Internal noise refers to the fact that neural responses are noisy. For example, a doctor may see many tumors a day and as such develop a set of neurons used when making decisions on whether a scan shows a tumor. These hypothetical tumor detectors will give noisy and variable responses. After one glance at a scan of a healthy lung, the hypothetical tumor detectors might fire 10 spikes per second. After a different glance at the same scan and under the same conditions, these neurons might fire 40 spikes per second.

Internal response: It is actually not likely that there are tumor detector neurons in a radiologist's brain. But there is some internal state, reflected by neural activity somewhere in the brain, that determines the doctor's impression about whether a tumor is present. This is a fundamental issue; the state of the doctor's mind is reflected by neural activity somewhere in her brain. This neural activity might be concentrated in just a few neurons, or it might be distributed across a large number of neurons. Since we do not know much about where/when this neural activity is, let's simply refer to it as the doctor's *internal response*.

This internal response is inherently noisy. Even when there is no tumor present (no-signal trials), there will be some internal response (sometimes more, sometimes less) in the doctor's sensory system.

52. Which of the following does this passage refer to?
   a. Sensory adaptation
   b. Signal detection theory
   c. Somatosensory system
   d. Weber's law

53. The doctor's neural activity in the brain is an example of which of the following?
   a. Internal noise
   b. External noise
   c. Internal response
   d. Uncertainty

54. The branch of psychology that deals with the relationships between physical stimuli (i.e., the film) and mental phenomena (i.e., the doctor's internal processing of what is seen on the film) is which of the following?
   a. Psychophysics
   b. Gestalt psychology
   c. Neuroscience
   d. Cognitive psychology

55. Two sets of doctors (first-year residents and attending physicians) were compared based on their resulting outcomes for a set of radiological images using experimental design. If the attending physicians were the control group, what were the first-year residents?
   a. The dependent variable
   b. The independent variable
   c. The experimental group
   d. The treatment group

56. Which of the following quotes from the passage is an example of neuroscience?
   a. "This internal response is inherently noisy. Even when there is no tumor present (no-signal trials), there will be some internal response (sometimes more, sometimes less) in the doctor's sensory system."
   b. "Detecting a tumor is difficult, and there will always be some amount of uncertainty."
   c. "Or there can be something in the person's lung that is fine but looks a bit like a tumor."
   d. "But there is some internal state, reflected by neural activity somewhere in the brain, that determines the doctor's impression about whether a tumor is present."

57. A prisoner who has been in solitary confinement is released back into the general population four days early due to good behavior. Which type of conditioning is being used in this case?
   a. Extinction
   b. Classical conditioning
   c. Negative reinforcement
   d. Positive reinforcement

58. An adult who has a caregiver, such as a family member, is exhibiting signs of withdrawal from social activities, lack of alertness, bruises, and frequent arguments with his caregiver. He is MOST likely exhibiting signs of
  a. multiple sclerosis.
  b. elder abuse.
  c. Parkinson's disease.
  d. Alzheimer's disease.

59. Which of the following BEST takes the view that people become criminals when characterized as such and when they accept the characterization as a personal identity?
  a. Differential association
  b. Strain theory
  c. Labeling theory
  d. Behaviorism

Part 4: Critical Analysis and Reasoning Skills

53 Questions
90 Minutes

Use the following passage to answer questions 1 through 6.

(1)   In order to understand the social and dynamic significance of modern dramatic art it is necessary, I believe, to ascertain the difference between the functions of art for art's sake and art as the mirror of life.

(2)   Art for art's sake presupposes an attitude of aloofness on the part of the artist toward the complex struggle of life: he must rise above the ebb and tide of life. He is to be merely an artistic conjurer of beautiful forms, a creator of pure fancy.

(3)   That is not the attitude of modern art, which is preeminently the reflex, the mirror of life. The artist, being a part of life, cannot detach himself from the events and occurrences that pass panorama-like before his eyes, impressing themselves upon his emotional and intellectual vision.

(4)   The modern artist is, in the words of August Strindberg, "a lay preacher popularizing the pressing questions of his time." Not necessarily because his aim is to proselytize, but because he can best express himself by being true to life.

(5)   Millet, Meunier, Turgenev, Dostoyevsky, Emerson, Walt Whitman, Tolstoy, Ibsen, Strindberg, Hauptmann and a host of others mirror in their work as much of the spiritual and social revolt as is expressed by the most fiery speech of the propagandist. And more important still, they compel far greater attention. Their creative genius, imbued with

the spirit of sincerity and truth, strikes root where the ordinary word often falls on barren soil.

(6) The reason that many radicals as well as conservatives fail to grasp the powerful message of art is perhaps not far to seek. The average radical is as hidebound by mere terms as the man devoid of all ideas. "Bloated plutocrats," "economic determinism," "class consciousness," and similar expressions sum up for him the symbols of revolt. But since art speaks a language of its own, a language embracing the entire gamut of human emotions, it often sounds meaningless to those whose hearing has been dulled by the din of stereotyped phrases.

(7) On the other hand, the conservative sees danger only in the advocacy of the Red Flag. He has too long been fed on the historic legend that it is only the "rabble" which makes revolutions, and not those who wield the brush or pen. It is therefore legitimate to applaud the artist and hound the rabble. Both radical and conservative have to learn that any mode of creative work, which with true perception portrays social wrongs earnestly and boldly, may be a greater menace to our social fabric and a more powerful inspiration than the wildest harangue of the soapbox orator.

(8) Unfortunately, we in America have so far looked upon the theater as a place of amusement only, exclusive of ideas and inspiration. Because the modern drama of Europe has until recently been inaccessible in printed form to the average theatergoer in this country, he had to content himself with the interpretation, or rather misinterpretation, of our dramatic critics. As a result the social significance of the Modern Drama has well nigh been lost to the general public.

—Emma Goldman, *The Social Significance of the Modern Drama*

1. The passage's central thesis is that
   a. modern European drama is superior to modern American drama.
   b. radical and conservative political thinkers need more creativity.
   c. modern drama has the power to evoke political change.
   d. art for art's sake is an aesthetic movement devoid of meaning.

2. What is the closest meaning of the phrase "soapbox orator" (paragraph 7)?
   a. A person who gives improvised political speeches
   b. A person of short stature who needs to stand on a box to get attention
   c. A person whose eloquence is considered pure
   d. A person who advocates the need for cleanliness in society

3. Emma Goldman's statement about how European drama has been "inaccessible in printed form" (paragraph 8) to the average American theatergoer most likely implies that
   a. Goldman wrote this before the advent of the Internet.
   b. Americans never travel to Europe to see great theater.
   c. Americans have yet to experience the power of a political message in dramatic art.
   d. the average American would rather attend the theater than read a play.

4. Goldman uses the phrases "bloated plutocrats," "economic determinism," and "class consciousness" (paragraph 6) in order to
   a. enumerate the ideals that ought to be the true cause of art.
   b. provide examples of phrases that discuss social revolt but do not stir emotion.
   c. show examples of the symbolism of revolt in the plays of Strindberg.
   d. provide examples of phrases that are devoid of ideas.

5. The painter James McNeill Whistler once wrote, "Art should be independent of all claptrap—should stand alone, and appeal to the artistic sense of eye or ear, without confounding this with emotions entirely foreign to it, as devotion, pity, love, patriotism, and the like." Based on the passage, which of the following statements most closely resembles how the author would respond to Whistler?
   a. Emotion isn't foreign to art; in fact, it is an inherent quality in the language of modern art.
   b. The artist's intention is irrelevant; the viewer decides the message.
   c. Dramatic art is more complex than painting and usually has something to say about life.
   d. Radical and conservative politicians should be independent of all clap-trap.

6. According to the passage, which of the following would have the most effective political message?
   a. A bumper sticker that contains the poet Walt Whitman's phrase "Resist much, obey little."
   b. A television advertisement that includes famous Broadway actors
   c. A sermon by Dr. Martin Luther King, Jr.
   d. A painting by Banksy, the graffiti artist/political activist

Use the following passage to answer questions 7 through 12.

(1) Since Gertrude Stein's work was first brought to my attention I have been thinking of it as the most important pioneer work done in the field of letters in my time. The loud guffaws of the general public that must inevitably follow the bringing forward of more of her work do not irritate me but I would like it if writers, and particularly young writers, would come to understand a little what she is trying to do and what she is in my opinion doing.

(2)   My thought in the matter is something like this—that every artist working with words as his medium, must at times be profoundly irritated by what seems the limitations of his medium. What things does he not wish to create with words! There is the mind of the reader before him and he would like to create in that reader's mind a whole new world of sensations, or rather one might better say he would like to call back into life all of the dead and sleeping senses.

(3)   There is a thing one might call "the extension of the province of his art" one wants to achieve. One works with words and one would like words that have a taste on the lips, that have a perfume to the nostrils, rattling words one can throw into a box and shake, making a sharp, jingling sound, words that, when seen on the printed page, have a distinct arresting effect upon the eye, words that when they jump out from under the pen one may feel with the fingers as one might caress the cheeks of his beloved.

(4)   And what I think is that these books of Gertrude Stein's do in a very real sense recreate life in words.

(5)   We writers are, you see, all in such a hurry. There are such grand things we must do. For one thing the Great American Novel must be written and there is the American or English Stage that must be uplifted by our very important contributions, to say nothing of the epic poems, sonnets to my lady's eyes, and whatnot. We are all busy getting these grand and important thoughts and emotions into the pages of printed books.

(6)   And in the meantime the little words, that are the soldiers with which we great generals must make our conquests, are neglected.

(7)   There is a city of English and American words and it has been a neglected city. Strong broad shouldered words, that should be marching across open fields under the blue sky, are clerking in little dusty dry goods stores, young virgin words are being allowed to consort with whores, learned words have been put to the ditch digger's trade. Only yesterday I saw a word that once called a whole nation to arms serving in the mean capacity of advertising laundry soap.

(8)   For me the work of Gertrude Stein consists in a rebuilding, an entire new recasting of life, in the city of words. Here is one artist who has been able to accept ridicule, who has even forgone the privilege of writing the great American novel, uplifting our English speaking stage, and wearing the bays of the great poets, to go live among the little housekeeping words, the swaggering bullying street-corner words, the honest working, money saving words, and all the other forgotten and neglected citizens of the sacred and half forgotten city.

—Sherwood Anderson, foreword to *Geography and Plays* by Gertrude Stein

7. Which of the following choices best explain what Sherwood Anderson means by the statement that Stein lives among "the little housekeeping words, the swaggering bullying street-corner words"?
   a. She is not paid well for her writing.
   b. She writes in plain yet forceful everyday language.
   c. She writes about subjects like street bullying and housekeeping.
   d. She is the voice of the downtrodden.

8. Judging from the context, the "loud guffaws" that Anderson refers to in paragraph 1 most likely imply that
   a. the general public would be delighted to read more of Stein's work.
   b. the general public mocks Stein's work because they do not understand its significance.
   c. Stein writes comical poems.
   d. Stein writes for writers and not the general public.

9. Anderson discusses a writer's irritation with the "limitations of his medium" (paragraph 2) most likely to emphasize that
   a. writing is difficult on its own but Stein also has to endure criticism of her work.
   b. Stein breaks the limitations of the medium by recasting plain words in a new way.
   c. Stein's work cannot accurately be captured in prose.
   d. multimedia work would create a more complex literature in society.

10. Based on the information in the passage, which of the following lines of poetry most closely match Anderson's description of Gertrude Stein's work?
   a. "Apple plum, carpet steak, seed clam, colored wine, calm seen, cold cream."
   b. "My mistress' eyes are nothing like the sun; Coral is far more red than her lips' red."
   c. "Keep, ancient lands, your storied pomp!" cries she with silent lips. "Give me your tired, your poor, your huddled masses yearning to breathe free."
   d. "Exultation is the going of an inland soul to sea—Past the houses, past the headlands, Into deep eternity!"

11. Which of the following criticisms of Stein might Anderson be responding to?
   a. Stein's poetry is just a lot of words strung together, omitting sentence structure, omitting sense—it is like a facile grocery list.
   b. Stein's poetry suffers because of its overuse of rhyme and formal gimmicks.
   c. Stein's poetry mixes high and low cultures, the elegant and the vulgar; it is a mongrel.
   d. Stein's poetry relies too heavily on the Romantics.

12. Based on the information in the passage, with which of the following attitudes in literary criticism is Sherwood Anderson most likely to agree?
   a. In order to truly understand a writer's poetry, the reader must know something about the poet's life.
   b. A poem does not require beauty, meaning, or any traditional structure, but it should be an experience of language for its reader.
   c. The reader must make meaning out of a poem, regardless of the poet's intended meaning.
   d. In order to understand the meaning of a poem, the reader has to closely examine its structure.

Use the following passage to answer questions 13 through 18.

(1) Authors of the highest eminence seem to be fully satisfied with the view that each species has been independently created. To my mind it accords better with what we know of the laws impressed on matter by the Creator, that the production and extinction of the past and present inhabitants of the world should have been due to secondary causes, like those determining the birth and death of the individual. When I view all beings not as special creations, but as the lineal descendants of some few beings which lived long before the first bed of the Silurian system was deposited, they seem to me to become ennobled. Judging from the past, we may safely infer that not one living species will transmit its unaltered likeness to a distant futurity. And of the species now living very few will transmit progeny of any kind to a far distant futurity; for the manner in which all organic beings are grouped, shows that the greater number of species of each genus, and all

the species of many genera, have left no descendants, but have become utterly extinct. We can so far take a prophetic glance into futurity as to foretell that it will be the common and widely-spread species, belonging to the larger and dominant groups, which will ultimately prevail and procreate new and dominant species. As all the living forms of life are the lineal descendants of those which lived long before the Silurian epoch, we may feel certain that the ordinary succession by generation has never once been broken, and that no cataclysm has desolated the whole world. Hence we may look with some confidence to a secure future of equally inappreciable length. And as natural selection works solely by and for the good of each being, all corporeal and mental endowments will tend to progress towards perfection.

(2) It is interesting to contemplate an entangled bank, clothed with many plants of many kinds, with birds singing on the bushes, with various insects flitting about, and with worms crawling through the damp earth, and to reflect that these elaborately constructed forms, so different from each other, and dependent on each other in so complex a manner, have all been produced by laws acting around us. These laws, taken in the largest sense, being Growth with Reproduction; Inheritance which is almost implied by reproduction; Variability from the indirect and direct action of the external conditions of life, and from use and disuse; a Ratio of Increase so high as to lead to a Struggle for Life, and as a consequence to Natural Selection, entailing Divergence of Character and the Extinction of less-improved forms. Thus, from the war of nature, from famine and death, the most exalted object which we are capable of

conceiving, namely, the production of the higher animals, directly follows. There is grandeur in this view of life, with its several powers, having been originally breathed into a few forms or into one; and that, whilst this planet has gone cycling on according to the fixed law of gravity, from so simple a beginning endless forms most beautiful and most wonderful have been, and are being, evolved.
—Charles Darwin, *Origin of Species*

13. Which of the following best captures the main goal of the passage?
   a. To dispute authors who view species as having been independently created
   b. To describe the effects of gravity over time on various species
   c. To portray the beauty and perfection of all living things
   d. To theorize how the multitude of life as it presently exists on the planet arose

14. Darwin's use of the words "ennobled" (first paragraph) and "grandeur" (second paragraph) is most likely an attempt to
   a. suggest all living beings originated from divine creation.
   b. highlight that nature is a product of savagery in the survival of the fittest.
   c. advocate that all living forms currently in existence are in their most perfect state.
   d. emphasize a sense of awe for the intricacies and interplay inherent in the process of evolution.

15. "Thus, from the war of nature, from famine and death, the most exalted object which we are capable of conceiving, namely, the production of the higher animals, directly follows."

Which is the most logical implication of this passage excerpt?

   a. Humankind is not capable of conceiving a being greater than itself.
   b. There is irony in natural selection because good things arise from bad.
   c. The most exalted object we are capable of conceiving is a predator.
   d. War in human society is perfectly natural and is a product of evolution.

16. If Darwin had been aware of contemporary genetic science, he would most likely agree that futurity would contain species that arise from which of the following?
   a. The work of scientists in the field of genetic modification who seek to create a more perfect species
   b. Mutations in the DNA of embryos that lead to radical transformations in the species' appearance or abilities
   c. Only large and dominant species that share DNA with current predator species like lions and sharks
   d. A new set of species that develop through small genetic variance in genomes from present-day species over many generations

17. If, as Richard Dawkins proposes in *The Selfish Gene*, ideas propagate in society and evolve by a process of natural selection, then which of the following statements is best supported by the description of the process of natural selection within the passage?
   a. Ideas are independently created within the brain of an individual.
   b. Weak ideas fall into disuse as stronger ideas win out and are reproduced throughout society.
   c. We can infer from ideas in the past that no currently accepted ideas will survive in the far-distant future.
   d. All ideas are descended from one or a few original ideas.

18. Which of the assertions regarding endangered species is a statement with which Darwin would most probably agree?
   a. The protection of endangered species is one of society's most important moral obligations.
   b. Endangered species are a rare and beautiful byproduct of natural selection.
   c. Species that are endangered today will not likely survive to a distant future.
   d. Human interference with the natural world is the main cause of endangered species.

Use the following passage to answer questions 19 through 24.

(1)   It is said that Mirabeau took to highway robbery "to ascertain what degree of resolution was necessary in order to place one's self in formal opposition to the most sacred laws of society." He declared that "a soldier who fights in the ranks does not require half so much courage as a footpad"—"that honor and religion have never stood in the way of a

well-considered and a firm resolve." This was manly, as the world goes; and yet it was idle, if not desperate. A saner man would have found himself often enough "in formal opposition" to what are deemed "the most sacred laws of society," through obedience to yet more sacred laws, and so have tested his resolution without going out of his way. It is not for a man to put himself in such an attitude to society, but to maintain himself in whatever attitude he find himself through obedience to the laws of his being, which will never be one of opposition to a just government, if he should chance to meet with such.

(2)   I left the woods for as good a reason as I went there. Perhaps it seemed to me that I had several more lives to live, and could not spare any more time for that one. It is remarkable how easily and insensibly we fall into a particular route, and make a beaten track for ourselves. I had not lived there a week before my feet wore a path from my door to the pond-side; and though it is five or six years since I trod it, it is still quite distinct. It is true, I fear, that others may have fallen into it, and so helped to keep it open. The surface of the earth is soft and impressible by the feet of men; and so with the paths which the mind travels. How worn and dusty, then, must be the highways of the world, how deep the ruts of tradition and conformity! I did not wish to take a cabin passage, but rather to go before the mast and on the deck of the world, for there I could best see the moonlight amid the mountains. I do not wish to go below now.

(3)   I learned this, at least, by my experiment: that if one advances confidently in the direction of his dreams, and endeavors to live the life which he has imagined, he will meet with a success unexpected in common hours. He will put some things behind, will pass an invisible

boundary; new, universal, and more liberal laws will begin to establish themselves around and within him; or the old laws be expanded, and interpreted in his favor in a more liberal sense, and he will live with the license of a higher order of beings. In proportion as he simplifies his life, the laws of the universe will appear less complex, and solitude will not be solitude, nor poverty, nor weakness. If you have built castles in the air, your work need not be lost; that is where they should be. Now put the foundations under them.

—Henry David Thoreau, *Walden: Or Life in the Woods*

19. Which of the following best captures the main goal of Thoreau in this passage?
    a. To dissect Mirabeau's flawed reasoning when it comes to society's most sacred laws
    b. To explain the author's personal reasons for leaving the woods for a sea voyage
    c. To point out that a government that is just is a rarity and that therefore laws are rarely just
    d. To emphasize that one should be governed by one's own personal truth

20. When Thoreau writes "The surface of the earth is soft and impressible by the feet of men; and so with the paths which the mind travels," the earth metaphor mostly likely implies that
    a. people do not often think outside the box because they evolved on a soft earth.
    b. minds are impressionable, malleable, and subject to conformity.
    d. neural pathways in the brain do not differ much between different societies.
    d. men who follow traditions have soft minds.

21. Mirabeau was an early leader of the French Revolution. Thoreau employs Mirabeau's quote, "a soldier who fights in the ranks does not require half so much courage as a footpad,"* in order to argue that

*A footpad is a thief who robs pedestrians.

  a. militaries can be used for cowardly and nefarious purposes.
  b. Mirabeau created an apt metaphor because footpads are not courageous.
  c. one ought not be defined by his acts of disobedience to others but by his obedience to the laws of his own nature.
  d. being told what to do and following orders do not require courage.

22. Based on the discussion in the first paragraph of the passage, Thoreau would most likely agree with which of the following acts of disobedience?
  a. A civil rights activist's refusal to give up her seat on a bus, in defiance of segregation laws
  b. A hungry man's decision to steal a loaf of bread
  c. A driver who disobeys the speed limit because he enjoys going fast
  d. A banker's exploitation of loopholes in financial laws

23. Based on Thoreau's attitudes as expressed in the passage, if he were to go on a sea voyage, he would most likely perform which of the following actions?
  a. Revel in the sights and experiences of the voyage
  b. Disobey the captain's orders and climb the ship's mast just to show his resolve
  c. Stay below deck and keep to himself
  d. Jump ship because it is unconventional

24. Based on the information in the passage, with which of the following statements about the individual would Thoreau most likely agree?
  a. The individual begins as a blank slate and is shaped by experience.
  b. The individual is a collection of chemicals subject to his or her own DNA.
  c. The individual must create his or her own value system rather than follow an external socially imposed code.
  d. The individual as a whole is an illusion but actually consists of distinct yet interconnected thought processes.

Use the following passage to answer questions 25 through 30.

When one has been wandering for a whole morning through a valley of perfect silence, where everything around, which is motionless, is colossal, and everything which has motion, resistless; where the strength and the glory of nature are principally developed in the very forces which feed upon her majesty; and where, in the midst of mightiness which seems imperishable, all that is indeed eternal is the influence of desolation; one is apt to be surprised, and by no means agreeably, to find, crouched behind some projecting rock, a piece of architecture which is neat in the extreme, though in the midst of wildness, weak in the midst of strength, contemptible in the midst of immensity. There is something offensive in its neatness: for the wood is almost always perfectly clean, and looks as if it had just been cut; it is consequently raw in its color, and destitute of all variety of tone. This is especially disagreeable, when the eye has been previously accustomed to, and finds, everywhere around, the exquisite mingling of color, and confused, though perpetually graceful, forms, by which the details of mountain scenery are peculiarly distinguished. Every fragment of rock is finished in its effect, tinted with thousands of pale lichens and fresh mosses; every pine tree is warm with the life of various vegetation; every grassy bank glowing with mellowed color, and waving with delicate leafage. How, then, can the contrast be otherwise than painful, between this perfect loveliness, and the dead, raw, lifeless surface of the deal boards of the cottage. Its weakness is pitiable; for, though there is always evidence of considerable strength on close examination, there is no effect of strength: the real thickness of the logs is concealed by the cutting and carving of their exposed surfaces; and even what is seen is felt to be so utterly contemptible, when opposed to the destructive forces which are in operation around, that the feelings are irritated at the imagined audacity of the inanimate object, with the self-conceit of its impotence; and, finally, the eye is offended at its want of size. It does not, as might be at first supposed, enhance the sublimity of surrounding scenery by its littleness, for it provokes no comparison; and there must be proportion between objects, or they cannot be compared. If the Parthenon, or the Pyramid of Cheops, or St. Peter's, were placed in the same situation, the mind would first form a just estimate of the magnificence of the building, and then be trebly impressed with the size of the masses which overwhelmed it. The architecture would not lose, and the crags would gain, by the juxtaposition; but the cottage, which must be felt to be a thing which the weakest stream of the Alps could toss down before it like a foam-globe, is offensively contemptible: it is like a child's toy let fall accidentally on the hillside; it does not unite with the scene; it is not content to sink into a quiet corner, and personify humility and peace; but it draws attention upon itself by its pretension to decoration, while its decorations themselves cannot bear examination, because they are useless, unmeaning and incongruous.

—John Ruskin, *Poetry of Architecture*

25. What is the passage's central thesis?
   a. Neatness in architecture is contemptible.
   b. Architecture should be in harmony with its surroundings.
   c. The stamp of human civilization on nature is offensive.
   d. A beautiful piece of architecture cannot compare to the beauty of nature.

26. Judging from the context, the phrase "it is like a child's toy let fall accidentally on the hillside" most likely implies that
   a. the cottage is dilapidated and in need of repair.
   b. the creator of the cottage was not a serious architect.
   d. the cottage looks very small and out of place.
   d. viewers have a wondrous childlike fascination with the cottage.

27. Ruskin mentions the Parthenon, the Pyramid of Cheops, and St. Peter's in order to show that
   a. the magnitude of the Alps can only be matched by a magnificent building.
   b. great architecture is more likely found in cities.
   c. there has been a decline in modern architecture.
   d. buildings made of stone are more lasting and pleasing to the eye than wood construction.

28. Which of the following buildings would Ruskin consider offensive, according to his views as expressed in the passage?
   a. A McDonald's in Times Square
   b. A skyscraper at the end of a country lane
   c. Pyramids in the desert
   d. A castle in the Alps

29. Which of the following statements would Ruskin most likely offer as advice to an architect early in his career?
   a. Have thick skin because your architecture will be criticized.
   b. Do not treat your architectural projects like children's toys.
   c. Do not build cottages on hillsides.
   d. Create buildings that harmonize with their surroundings.

30. Based on the discussion in the passage, which of the following statements made by famed architect Frank Lloyd Wright would Ruskin most closely agree with?
   a. "All artistic creation has its own philosophy. It is the first condition of creation."
   b. "No house should ever be *on* a hill or *on* anything. It should be *of* the hill. Belonging to it. Hill and house should live together each the happier for the other."
   c. "All materials may be beautiful, their beauty much or entirely depending upon how well they are used by the architect."
   d. "A wood building will look like none other, for it will glorify the stick. A steel and glass building could not possibly look like anything but itself. It will glorify steel and glass."

Use the following passage to answer questions 31 through 36.

(1) Freud's theories are anything but theoretical. He was moved by the fact that there always seemed to be a close connection between his patients' dreams and their mental abnormalities, to collect thousands of dreams and to compare them with the case histories in his possession. He did not start out with a preconceived bias, hoping to find evidence which might support his views. He looked at facts a thousand times "until they began to tell him something." His attitude toward dream study was, in other words, that of a statistician who does not know, and has no means of foreseeing, what conclusions will be forced on him by the information he is gathering, but who is fully prepared to accept those unavoidable conclusions.

(2) This was indeed a novel way in psychology. Psychologists had always been wont to build, in what Bleuler calls "autistic ways," that is through methods in no ways supported by evidence, some attractive hypothesis, which sprung from their brain, like Minerva from Jove's brain, fully armed. After which, they would stretch upon that unyielding frame the hide of a reality which they had previously killed. It is only to minds suffering from the same distortions, to minds also autistically inclined, that those empty, artificial structures appear acceptable molds for philosophic thinking. The pragmatic view that "truth is what works" had not been as yet expressed when Freud published his revolutionary views on the psychology of dreams.

(3) Five facts of first magnitude were made obvious to the world by his interpretation of dreams. First of all, Freud pointed out a constant connection between some part of every dream and some detail of the dreamer's

life during the previous waking state. This positively establishes a relation between sleeping states and waking states and disposes of the widely prevalent view that dreams are purely nonsensical phenomena coming from nowhere and leading nowhere. Secondly, Freud, after studying the dreamer's life and modes of thought, after noting down all his mannerisms and the apparently insignificant details of his conduct which reveal his secret thoughts, came to the conclusion that there was in every dream the attempted or successful gratification of some wish, conscious or unconscious. Thirdly, he proved that many of our dream visions are symbolical, which causes us to consider them as absurd and unintelligible; the universality of those symbols, however, makes them very transparent to the trained observer. Fourthly, Freud showed that sexual desires play an enormous part in our unconscious, a part which puritanical hypocrisy has always tried to minimize, if not to ignore entirely. Finally, Freud established a direct connection between dreams and insanity, between the symbolic visions of our sleep and the symbolic actions of the mentally deranged. There were, of course, many other observations which Freud made while dissecting the dreams of his patients, but not all of them present as much interest as the foregoing nor were they as revolutionary or likely to wield as much influence on modern psychiatry.

(4)   Other explorers have struck the path blazed by Freud leading into man's unconscious. Jung of Zurich, Adler of Vienna and Kempf of Washington, D.C., have made to the study of the unconscious, contributions which have brought that study into fields which Freud himself never dreamt of invading. One fact which cannot be too emphatically stated, however, is that but for Freud's wish fulfillment theory of dreams, neither Jung's "energic theory," nor Adler's theory of "organ inferiority and compensation," nor Kempf's "dynamic mechanism" might have been formulated. Freud is the father of modern abnormal psychology and he established the psychoanalytical point of view.

—Andre Tridon, introduction to Freud's *Dream Psychology: Psychoanalysis for Beginners*

31. According to the passage, which of the following statements accord with Freud's theories of dream psychology?

> I. Dreams fulfill a wish, whether the sleeper is aware of that wish or not.
> II. Symbolic actions in sleep mirror symbolic actions of the insane.
> III. Dreams are made up of symbols whose meaning may not be apparent to the dreamer.

a. I only
b. III only
c. I and II only
d. I, II, and III

32. Judging from the context, the term "autistic ways" (paragraph 2) most likely refers to the psychologists' methods as
a. characterized by emotional detachment.
b. plagued by impaired communication.
c. not based on observed information.
d. shortsighted and narcissistic.

33. Which of the following best expresses the relationship between the reference to the Roman goddess Minerva and the stretched "hide of a reality" (paragraph 2)?
- **a.** Minerva, the goddess of war, kills by skinning her victims.
- **b.** The "birth" of some psychologists' theories led to the "death" of reality.
- **c.** Psychologists considered themselves godlike, so reality was open to interpretation.
- **d.** An idea can spring from the brain with full force but gets weakened upon further reflection.

34. Which of the following is the most incisive criticism of Tridon's statement that Freud "looked at facts a thousand times 'until they began to tell him something'"?
- **a.** This statement is unconvincing because it does not appeal to the reader's emotions.
- **b.** The statement is unconvincing because the author is trying to defend Freud by quoting Freud himself.
- **c.** This statement is unconvincing because it still sounds like Freud could have made up his whole theory.
- **d.** This statement is unconvincing because the phrase "a thousand times" is not literally true, sounds unspecific, and does not seem like a factual piece of evidence.

35. Which of the following statements critical of Freud does the opening paragraph of the passage most nearly respond to?
- **a.** Freud's personal concern with his own dreams of castration caused him to search for evidence of sexual sublimation in his patients' dreams.
- **b.** Interpretation of dream symbols was not invented by Freud; in fact, not much of his dream theory can be called original.
- **c.** Freud did not accept any criticism of his work and he is therefore unscientific.
- **d.** Freud frequently used cocaine for migraines, which affected his ability to accurately interpret the facts of his patients' ailments.

36. If three people all wake up from similar dreams of being late for a meeting and finding that they are naked when they get there, which of the following statements is the most logical conclusion to make according to Freud's theories as outlined in the passage?
- **a.** The three dreamers all suffer from the same mental disorder.
- **b.** The three dreamers all have an unconscious wish to be exhibitionists.
- **c.** The three dreamers are all having similar conflicts in their daily lives.
- **d.** The three dreamers are psychically connected to each other.

Use the following passage to answer questions 37 through 41.

(1) The first glimpse we have that the Greeks possessed an idea of the shape of the earth comes from the poems of Homer. These poems show an intimate knowledge of Northern Greece and of the western coasts of Asia Minor, some acquaintance with Egypt, Cyprus, and Sicily; but all the rest, even of the Eastern

Mediterranean, is only vaguely conceived by their author. Where he does not know he imagines, and some of his imaginings have had a most important influence upon the progress of geographical knowledge. Thus he conceives of the world as being a sort of flat shield, with an extremely wide river surrounding it, known as Ocean. The center of this shield was at Delphi, which was regarded as the "navel" of the inhabited world. According to Hesiod, who came after Homer, up in the far north were placed a people known as the Hyperboreani, or those who dwelt at the back of the north wind; while a corresponding place in the south was taken by the Abyssinians. All these four conceptions had an important influence on the views that men had of the world. Homer also mentioned the pygmies living in Africa. These were regarded as fabulous, until they were re-discovered by Dr. Schweinfurth and Mr. Stanley in the late 19th century.

(2)   It is probable that the Greeks obtained the idea of an all-encircling ocean from the Babylonians. Inhabitants of Mesopotamia would find themselves reaching the ocean in almost any direction in which they travelled— either the Caspian, the Black Sea, the Mediterranean, or the Persian Gulf. Accordingly, the oldest map of the world which has been found is one with a cuneiform inscription, that represents the plain of Mesopotamia with the Euphrates flowing through it, surrounded by two concentric circles, which are named "briny waters." Outside these, however, are seven detached islets, possibly representing the seven zones or climates into which the world was divided according to the ideas of the Babylonians. What was roughly true of Babylonia did not in any way match the geographical position of Greece, and it is therefore probable that they obtained

their ideas of the surrounding ocean from the Babylonians.

(3)   It was after the period of Homer and Hesiod that the first great expansion of Greek knowledge about the world began, through extensive colonization which was carried out by the Greeks around the Eastern Mediterranean. Even to this day the natives of the southern part of Italy speak a Greek dialect, owing to the wide extent of Greek colonies in that country, which used to be called "Magna Grecia," or "Great Greece." Marseilles was also one of the Greek colonies (600 B.C.), which, in its turn, sent out other colonies along the Gulf of Lyons. In the East, too, Greek cities were dotted along the coast of the Black Sea, one of which, Byzantium, was destined to be of world-historic importance. So, too, the Greeks created colonies in North Africa, and among the islands of the Aegean Sea throughout the sixth and fifth centuries B.C., and in almost every case communication was kept up between the colonies and the mother-country.

(4)   Now, the one quality which has made the Greeks so distinguished in the world's history was their curiosity; and it was natural that they should desire to know, and to put on record, the large amount of information brought to the mainland of Greece from the innumerable Greek colonies. But to record geographical knowledge, the first thing that is necessary is a map and accordingly, it is a Greek philosopher named Anaximander of Miletus, of the sixth century B.C., to whom we owe the invention of map-drawing.

—Joseph Jacobs, *The Story of Geographical Discovery: How the World Became Known*

37. What is the main purpose of this passage?
   a. To demonstrate the value of poetry as containing ancient truths
   b. To show that the Babylonians, not the Greeks, were the true inventors of mapmaking
   c. To denounce Greek colonization of the Eastern Mediterranean
   d. To trace the origins of geographical knowledge of the Greeks

38. Judging from the context, the "navel" mentioned in paragraph 1 could best be described as
   a. the location where Greek warships were stored.
   b. the lifeline that connected all Greek colonies.
   c. the central point of the world.
   d. the birthplace of the world.

39. The author mentions the discoveries of Dr. Schweinfurth and Mr. Stanley in order to strengthen his argument that
   a. fables in various cultures are often based on fact.
   b. countries may be discovered, but people cannot be.
   c. Homer was mistakenly credited for inventing pygmies.
   d. elements of geographical knowledge found in Homer's work are accurate.

40. Which of the following statements from the passage contradict the author's final sentence?
   a. "the oldest map of the world which has been found is one with a cuneiform inscription"
   b. "the one quality which has made the Greeks so distinguished in the world's history was their curiosity"
   c. "one of which, Byzantium, was destined to be of world-historic importance"
   d. "thus [Homer] conceives of the world as being a sort of flat shield, with an extremely wide river surrounding it, known as Ocean"

41. Based on the passage information, with which of the following statements about culture and geography is Jacobs most likely to agree?
   a. A war-like culture that colonizes foreign lands will undoubtedly have the greatest access to geographical information.
   b. The richest societies that have the ability to fund explorers will obtain the greatest geographical knowledge.
   c. The curious society that values knowledge will venture into the world and gain the greatest amount of geographical knowledge.
   d. A maritime culture is most likely to explore the farthest regions beyond its land and collect the greatest amount of geographical information.

Use the following passage to answer questions 42 through 47.

(1) In the search for certainty, it is natural to begin with our present experiences, and in some sense, no doubt, knowledge is to be derived from them. But any statement as to what it is that our immediate experiences make us know is very likely to be wrong. It seems to me that I am now sitting in a chair, at a table of a certain shape, on which I see sheets of paper with

writing or print. By turning my head I see out of the window buildings and clouds and the sun. I believe that the sun is about ninety-three million miles from the earth; that it is a hot globe many times bigger than the earth; that, owing to the earth's rotation, it rises every morning, and will continue to do so for an indefinite time in the future. I believe that, if any other normal person comes into my room, he will see the same chairs and tables and books and papers as I see, and that the table which I see is the same as the table which I feel pressing against my arm. All this seems to be so evident as to be hardly worth stating, except in answer to a man who doubts whether I know anything. Yet all this may be reasonably doubted, and all of it requires much careful discussion before we can be sure that we have stated it in a form that is wholly true.

(2)   To make our difficulties plain, let us concentrate attention on the table. To the eye it is oblong, brown and shiny, to the touch it is smooth and cool and hard; when I tap it, it gives out a wooden sound. Any one else who sees and feels and hears the table will agree with this description, so that it might seem as if no difficulty would arise; but as soon as we try to be more precise our troubles begin. Although I believe that the table is 'really' of the same color all over, the parts that reflect the light look much brighter than the other parts, and some parts look white because of reflected light. I know that, if I move, the parts that reflect the light will be different, so that the apparent distribution of colors on the table will change. It follows that if several people are looking at the table at the same moment, no two of them will see exactly the same distribution of colors, because no two can see it from exactly the same point of view, and any change in the point of view makes some change in the way the light is reflected.

(3)   For most practical purposes these differences are unimportant, but to the painter they are all-important: the painter has to unlearn the habit of thinking that things seem to have the color which common sense says they 'really' have, and to learn the habit of seeing things as they appear. Here we have already the beginning of one of the distinctions that cause most trouble in philosophy—the distinction between 'appearance' and 'reality,' between what things seem to be and what they are. The painter wants to know what things seem to be, the practical man and the philosopher want to know what they are; but the philosopher's wish to know this is stronger than the practical man's, and is more troubled by knowledge as to the difficulties of answering the question.

—Bertrand Russell, *Reason and Responsibility: Readings in Some Basic Problems of Philosophy*

42. What is the main purpose of this passage?
   a. To ascertain the true color of the table
   b. To explain the differences between painter's perceptions and philosopher's perceptions
   c. To discuss the difficulty in distinguishing appearance from reality
   d. To distinguish what is practical from what is fantastical

43. According to Russell, no two people will see the exact same color of the table at the same moment because
   a. there is no way of knowing whether what one person considers brown is the same as another's experience of the color.
   b. the psychological effect of color affects the viewer's perception.
   c. the light will reflect off the table differently from different viewpoints.
   d. people may be color blind, color deficient, or have other neural anomalies affecting their ability to distinguish color.

44. Russell's argument is most vulnerable to which of the following criticisms?

   a. He fails to consider the female perspective and therefore lacks an entirely different perception of reality.

   b. He fails to define "normal person," thus doubting perception but not the perceiver.

   c. His disbelief in his own senses must mean his judgment is impaired.

   d. He fails to consider quantum mechanics and the "imperceptible" reality of the table.

45. Russell references the precise distance from the earth to the sun (paragraph 1) most likely in order to

   a. foreshadow his discussion of how light reflects off a table in the next paragraph.

   b. show that even measurable scientific data is subject to perception.

   c. establish his awareness of scientific instruments that could enhance the naked eye and therefore create another view of the table.

   d. establish the differences between a normal perception and an enhanced perception like that of the painter's.

46. Considering Russell's assessment of the table's color, which of the following most closely resembles what he might say about the table's shape?

   a. The true shape of the table is indeterminable unless the viewer is an artist who has mastered perspective drawing.

   b. A practical human will have no interest in the shape of the table.

   c. The shape of the table will appear to change as the viewer walks around the room.

   d. Because the shape of the table can be determined through sight and touch, we can be more assured of its shape than its color.

47. Which of the following sentences, if added to the final paragraph, would contradict the author's arguments?

   I. In conclusion, any two people, whether painter or philosopher, will have similar perceptions of the table; they do not need to be exactly the same to determine that something really exists.

   II. The fact is, the human mind can consider a table from a myriad of perspectives.

   III. We therefore must conclude that a man can know something is true without requiring knowledge based on indisputable fact.

   IV. If we therefore cannot determine a table really exists, then nothing is certain, even the very concept of certainty.

   a. I and III only

   b. II only

   c. III only

   d. I, II, III, and IV

Use the following passage to answer questions 48 through 53.

(1)   In order to understand the meaning of *dialectical regeneration* we must first see clearly what we mean by dialect. We saw before that language has no independent substantial existence. Language exists in man, it lives in being spoken, it dies with each word that is pronounced, and is no longer heard. It is a mere accident that language should ever have been reduced to writing, and have been made the vehicle of a written literature. Even now the largest number of languages have produced no literature. Among the numerous tribes of Central Asia, Africa, America, and Polynesia, language still lives in its natural state, in a state of continual combustion; and it is there that we must go if we wish to gain an insight into the

growth of human speech previous to its being arrested by any literary interference.

(2)   What we are accustomed to call languages, the literary idioms of Greece, and Rome, and India, of Italy, France, and Spain, must be considered as artificial, rather than as natural forms of speech. The real and natural life of language is in its dialects, and in spite of the tyranny exercised by the classical or literary idioms, the day is still very far off which is to see the dialects, even of such classical languages as Italian and French, entirely eradicated. About twenty of the Italian dialects have been reduced to writing, and made known by the press. Champollion-Figeac reckons the most distinguishable dialects of France at fourteen. The number of modern Greek dialects is carried by some as high as seventy, and though many of these are hardly more than local varieties, yet some, like the Tzaconic, differ from the literary language as much as Doric differed from Attic. In the island of Lesbos, villages distant from each other not more than two or three hours have frequently peculiar words of their own, and their own peculiar pronunciation.

(3)   It is a mistake to imagine that dialects are everywhere corruptions of the literary language. Even in England, the local patois have many forms which are more primitive than the language of Shakespeare, and the richness of their vocabulary surpasses, on many points, that of the classical writers of any period. Dialects have always been the feeders rather than the channels of a literary language; anyhow, they are parallel streams which existed long before one of them was raised to that temporary eminence which is the result of literary cultivation.

(4)   What Grimm says of the origin of dialects in general applies only to such as are produced by phonetic corruption. "Dialects," he writes

"develop themselves progressively, and the more we look backward in the history of language the smaller is their number, and the less definite their features. All multiplicity arises gradually from an original unity." So it seems, indeed, if we build our theories of language exclusively on the materials supplied by literary idioms, such as Sanskrit, Greek, Latin, and Gothic. No doubt these are the royal heads in the history of language. But as political history ought to be more than a chronicle of royal dynasties, so the historian of language ought never to lose sight of those lower and popular strata of speech from which these dynasties originally sprang, and by which alone they are supported.

—Max Müller, *Lectures on the Science of Language*

48. Max Müller's description of a language that lives in a "continual state of combustion" most likely indicates that
  a. the language is dead.
  b. the language is constantly changing.
  c. the language is plagued by miscommunication.
  d. the language is explosive.

49. Which of the following phrases, as used in the passage, most suggests that Müller has a bias against the prominence of literary language?
  a. "independent, substantial existence" (paragraph 1)
  b. "tyranny" (paragraph 2)
  c. "the royal heads" (paragraph 4)
  d. "those lower and popular strata" (paragraph 4)

50. Grimm's argument, quoted in the final paragraph, is vulnerable to which of the following criticisms?
   a. The theory he posits is merely a copy of evolutionary theory: that all species sprung from one original.
   b. Given the small amount of evidence from ancient scrolls, it is impossible to determine a dialect's origins.
   c. The theory only applies to "corrupted dialects" stemming from languages with a written record.
   d. The theory does not take into account the copious number of dialects presently spoken.

51. Müller begins with the term *dialectical regeneration* but never explicitly defines it or returns to it. Given the rest of the passage discussion, which of the following most closely matches what he must mean by this phrase?
   a. The practice of transcribing dialects into a written form
   b. The growth of language through dialect
   c. The logic behind the rise to prominence of certain words
   d. The corruption of literary languages

52. Someone who agreed with Müller's characterization of how a language grows would most likely also agree with the idea that
   a. linguists should not study dead languages.
   b. linguists should not characterize languages as "corrupt."
   c. linguists should study languages that have no literature.
   d. linguists should not study literature.

53. Which of the following descriptions most closely matches how Müller conceives of dialects as discussed in the passage?
   a. A tree branch that grows out from a large central trunk
   b. A river in constant motion that feeds into and flows out of other rivers
   c. A rock that stands alone, firm and fixed in its place
   d. A sand grain, distinct yet indistinguishable from a larger whole

Answers

Part 1: Biological and Biochemical Foundations of Living Systems

1. a. The unit $k'_{NO, Ox}$, which represents NO scavenging activity, is the only parameter that directly correlates with the increase in MAP. The variants with high $k'_{NO, Ox}$ values are also associated with greater changes in MAP, suggesting that NO scavenging and depletion are responsible for hypertension. Neither low nor high P_{50} values, indicating high and low oxygen affinity, respectively, are associated with increases in MAP, while autoxidation, reflected by k_{autox}, could be due to unstable rHb dimers, but these values do not correlate with MAP increases.

2. c. The binding curve of hemoglobin for oxygen is sigmoidal because the protein can bind oxygen at high concentrations in lungs and release it at low concentrations in tissues. The mutants in choice **a** and **b** have high affinity for oxygen under both conditions, while the mutant in choice **d** has a low affinity for oxygen under both conditions.

3. b. It is critical to know the DNA sequence of a gene, specifically the cDNA (complementary DNA) sequence, to clone it. Expression of hemoglobin protein in bacteria is incorrect because recombinant hemoglobin has also been expressed in yeast (and expressed and purified from pigs). Additionally, the cDNA (complementary DNA) sequence is the sequence of the gene after splicing has occurred, so it is not necessary to know the splice donor and acceptor sites, and many genes are cloned and expressed without knowing their structure (although the crystal structure of hemoglobin was one of the first proteins to be solved, in the 1920s).

4. b. Blood transfusion can sometimes lead to increases in hemolysis, and thus extracellular levels of hemoglobin, but this generally occurs as a result of a rare allergic reaction. Hemolysis is a common complication of liver cirrhosis, inflammatory bowel disease, and malaria infection.

5. b. The pI of glutamic acid is 3.22 because it has two carboxyl groups (and one amino group). The other amino acids have only one carboxyl group (and one amino group) and consequently have similar pIs in the range of 6.0. (The pIs of alanine, glycine, and glutamine are 6.00, 5.97, and 5.65, respectively.)

6. b. Lysine is a charged amino acid, and charged amino acids usually cover the surface of the protein molecule. Isoleucine, alanine, and proline are hydrophobic amino acids, and hydrophobic amino acids are typically buried inside the core of the protein molecule.

7. d. Isoprene and myrcene are terpenes that do not contain oxygen. Terpenes are a type of hydrocarbon terpenoid that all have double bonds and are classified based on the number of 5-carbon units they contain (isoprene rule).

8. c. Certain lipids in bacterial and mammalian cell membranes are involved in intracellular and intercellular signaling. Cholesterol is not present in the membranes of prokaryotes, eukaryote cell membranes do not have negatively charged lipids on their surface, and bacterial plasma membranes are often made up of one main type of phospholipid, whereas the plasma membranes of most eukaryotes have a mixture of different phospholipids.

9. b. The rate of refolding is slower in the presence of MDH, as indicated by the lower amount of refolded Rho at the first five time points in the top four curves, but the concentration of refolded Rho at the last time point (60 min) is the same. The rate of refolding is slower in the presence of MDH, as indicated by the lower amount of refolded Rho at the first five time points in the top four curves. MDH transiently binds with the chaperones and competes with Rho. Additionally, the graph indicates that MDH does not form overly sticky complexes with the chaperones because they are still able to fold Rho, and the concentration of refolded Rho at the last time point (60 min), and thus the yield of refolded Rho, is the same in the presence of ATP (top two curves) whether MDH is present (solid circles) or absent (open circles).

10. d. Although phosphotidylinositol-3-kinase is regulated by chaperones, it does not have chaperone activity itself. (Isomerases with similar sounding names, peptidyl-prolyl *cis-trans* isomerase and protein disulfide isomerase), do have chaperone activity.) Hsp70 is one of the major chaperone families in eukaryotes. (In bacteria, it is called DnaK.) SecB is a soluble chaperone in bacteria, and GroEL/GroES is one of the major chaperone families in bacteria. (In eukaryotes, it is called Hsp60/Hsp10.) It should be easy to eliminate because it is the example in the passage.

11. a. Chaperones such as Hsp70 and GroEL can act iteratively on a molar excess of misfolded substrates. The passage states, "chaperones don't change the chemical composition of their misfolded polypeptide substrates," while, as stated in the passage, substrates may end up dissociating from the chaperone, and it should be clear that ATP is not required based on the graph; the refolding of Rho could occur, though to a lower level, in the absence of ATP (compare the middle two curves with the top two curves).

12. c. The passage states that cell stress, such as heat, can break weak bonds within a protein, particularly hydrogen bonds. Covalent bonds are the strongest bonds that are present in biochemicals; heat and denaturing agents do not break covalent bonds. Disulfide and carbon bonds are types of covalent bond; they are typically not disrupted by heat.

13. d. HEPES is an organic buffering agent that can actually increase protein stability and solubility. Urea is a denaturing agent that primarily disrupts the hydrogen bonds in a polypeptide, while extremes of pH, such as low (acids) or high (detergents), change the net charge on polypeptides and can alter electrostatic and hydrogen bonds, and alcohol destroys hydrogen bonds between the amide groups in the protein's secondary structure.

14. d. According to the model, GroEL has two subunits of hepatemeric rings, so there are 14 rings. If each ring binds to an ATP, there are 14 ATP molecules and thus 14 ADP molecules produced by ATP hydrolysis.

15. **a.** If an enzyme reacts by the two-step Michaelis-Menten mechanism, $V_{max} = k[E_t]$, where V_{max} is the maximum rate of the reaction, $[E_t]$ is the total concentration of enzyme, in this case chymotrypsin, and k is either the rate of enzyme-product complex formation or product release, whichever is lower (i.e., rate limiting). In this, as in most cases, the rate of product release, not the rate of enzyme-product complex formation, is limiting, so $V_{max} = 1.3 \times 10^{-4}/\text{sec} \times 2 \times 10^{-5}$ M. V_{max} is $\frac{1}{2} V_0$ only when the substrate concentration is equal to K_m for the reaction. In this case, the substrate concentration is not given.

16. **b.** In the plot for uncompetitive inhibition, the slope of the lines is the same for the different concentrations of inhibitor (methotrexate). In the plot for competitive inhibition, the slope increases as the concentration of inhibitor (methotrexate) increases and the lines intercept near 1/V, while the plot for mixed inhibition is similar to that of competitive inhibition, except the lines intercept before 1/V, and irreversible inhibition is a different category of inhibition (competitive, uncompetitive, and mixed are all types of reversible inhibition) in which the inhibitor binds covalently with or destroys an enzyme's functional group.

17. **c.** A competitive inhibitor binds to the active site of the enzyme and prevents the substrate from binding, whereas an uncompetitive inhibitor binds to a site distinct from the enzyme active site and only when the enzyme is in a complex with substrate.

18. **a.** The lower value of K_D corresponds with higher affinity of inhibitor for enzyme (in this case DHFR variants 1–4). 2.2 nM < 9.5 nM < 25 nM < 3×10^{-8} M (= 30 nM). These values are in the range of actual K_D for DHFR and MTX.

19. **a.** DNA strands anneal at physiological concentrations of pH and temperature, which is approximately 1 mM Mg^{2+} (and also the recommended concentration for PCR). It is recommended to increase the number of cycles and increase the DNA denaturation temperature to increase PCR yield and to maintain a balance of nucleotides to increase reaction fidelity.

20. **b.** The cell distinguishes the template and the newly synthesized strand, which is important for correct mismatches. Alkyl lesions on the nitrogen or oxygen of DNA damage the DNA, 5' phosphate groups are important for DNA ligation, and acetylation of histone groups plays a role in gene activation, not DNA repair.

21. **a.** According to the model of double-strand break repair for homologous genetic recombination, the 3' overhangs invade the homologous chromosome duplex, pairing with the complementary strand and displacing the other strand. The DSBs are repaired after this crossover event.

22. **c.** The DSB pattern for each strain, as indicated by the bands on the corresponding Southern blots, is similar. However, there are fewer bands for rad50+ at 5 and 6 hours than for rad50S and swi5Δ rhp57Δ, indicating that these mutants did not repair the DSB intermediates. The maximal level of DSBs is in the *rad50+* strain.

23. b. The detection of DNA by Southern blotting involves restriction enzyme digest to separate the DNA sample into fragments, separation of the fragments by gel electrophoresis, alkali treatment to denature the DNA, transfer of the DNA to a membrane, and then detection using a labeled (such as radiolabeled) DNA probe that is complementary to a repeat sequence in the DNA sample. If the amount of DNA sample is low, researchers can amplify the DNA using polymerase chain reaction, but this is not a necessary step.

24. d. Nucleotide probes can hybridize to RNA molecules if they contain complementary sequences and RNA can be separated by gel electrophoresis (although in a non-denaturing gel used for DNA, RNA molecules separate in an unpredictable smear). Although RNA cannot be directly amplified by polymerase chain reaction (it requires reverse transcription–polymerase chain reaction to produce cDNA), amplification is not a necessary step in Southern blotting. However, DNA can be harvested under conditions that do not recover RNA, including the use of enzymes that degrade RNA (RNAses).

25. c. Eukaryotic cells have two important types of repetitive DNA sequences: centromeres and telomeres. Only centromeres are required for the even distribution of chromosomes during mitosis; they link the chromosomes to spindles via microtubules. Telomeres do, however, play a role in the number of mitotic divisions a cell undergoes and in the recombination of homologous chromosomes during meiosis. Centromeres and telomeres are actually associated with transcriptionally inactive chromatin, also known as heterochromatin. The genomes of prokaryotes are typically circular and thus do not contain telomeres, whereas they do contain centromeres, which sometimes resemble eukaryotic centromeres.

26. c. F_{IS} is the inbreeding coefficient within populations, and it is zero if random mating occurs and high if inbreeding occurs. F_{IT} is a measure of gametes within an individual relative to the total population, and F_{ST} is a measure of random gametes within subpopulations. These values should be equal with each other to agree with the Hardy-Weinberg principle.

27. b. Based on the Hardy-Weinberg equation, the frequencies of the homozygous dominant allele (p^2), the homozygous recessive allele (q^2), and the heterozygous allele (pq) have to add up to 1 ($p^2 + q^2 + 2pq = 1$). In this case, $p^2 = 0.48$ (48%) and $q^2 = 0.36$ (36%), so $2pq = 0.16$ (16%).

28. c. The consensus gene promoter sequence in *E. coli* has an AT-rich region between positions −40 and −60 (relative to the transcription start site), followed by a TTGACA consensus sequence at −35 (which allows a high transcription rate), then a TATAAT, known as the Pribnow box, at −10.

29. c. According to Le Châtelier's principle, if a chemical reaction is at equilibrium, a change in conditions that displaces equilibrium will lead to a change toward a new equilibrium. Injection of $CO_2(g)$, which is a gas, would lead to a shift in the equilibrium from left to right, whereas injection of 2CO gas would lead to a shift from right to left. However, addition of C(s), which is a solid, does NOT lead to a shift in the reaction equilibrium if the pressure is kept constant because the concentration of a solid is independent of the amount present.

30. b. As stated in the passage, glucose is an aldose because it has a carbonyl group (C = O) at the end of its 6-carbon chain (at C1 in this chemical structure representation). Fructose belongs to the family of ketoses because its carbonyl group is within the carbon chain (at C2 in this chemical structure representation). Both glucose and fructose are hexoses, but the two families of monosaccharides are considered aldose and ketose.

31. c. As stated in the passage, glucose is an essential monosaccharide. It is one of eight essential monosaccharides that need to be obtained for proper functioning in humans, along with fucose, galactose, mannose, acetylglucosamine, acetylgalactosamine, xylose, and acetyl-neuraminic acid. (Although these sugars can be synthesized, it is more efficient to obtain them from diet.)

32. b. This choice is incorrect. As stated in the passage, tissues such as the lens, kidney, retina, and peripheral nerves have insulin-independent uptake of glucose. In contrast, insulin increases glucose uptake in adipose tissue.

33. d. Naphthalene is a compound with two benzene-like rings fused together. Analogs of naphthalene can have carbon in the place of nitrogen at some positions, as is the case for quinoline and purine. Cyclohexane is a single ring of six carbons with no double bonds, benzene is a single ring of six carbons with three double bonds, and anthracene is a compound with three benzene-like rings fused together.

34. b. As stated in the passage, IC_{50} corresponds to the drug concentration that is required to inhibit 50% of the activity of an enzyme, so the lower the IC_{50}, the more active the drug is against ALR2, which is the designated target. On the other hand, as stated in the passage, activity against ALR1 has been associated with adverse side effects, so the higher IC_{50} for ALR1 is desirable. The compound with the lowest IC_{50} for ALR2 and highest IC_{50} for ALR1 is compound 6.

35. a. Changes in compound color can be measured using spectrophotometry. Enzyme digest is a technique used for analyzing DNA, and gel electrophoresis is a technique for separating nucleic acids. Although color changes can be seen by microscopy, this technique is not necessarily quantitative, and electron microscopy is generally used for visualizing subcellular structures.

36. c. As stated in the passage, miRNAs are normally expressed in human cells (endogenous expression), whereas siRNAs are not normally expressed in human cells but can be introduced (exogenous expression). In terms of length, miRNAs are 21 to 23 nucleotides long and siRNAs are 22 nucleotides long, both miRNAs and siRNAs can block translation and degrade mRNAs, and both processed from their precursors—either miRNA precursors or dsRNAs—by Dicer.

37. b. As stated in the passage, lncRNAs often resemble mRNAs and are capped and polyadenylated. mRNAs also contain splice donor and acceptor sites, as do lncRNAs; however, mRNAs are not typically acetylated.

38. a. As stated in the text, miRNA molecules are 21 to 23 nucleotides, whereas lncRNA are long and resemble mRNAs. Sequence 1 is an miR122; sequence 2 is an lncRNA known as HOTTIP.

39. d. As stated in the text, "[s]everal properties of RNAs make them attractive clinical tools, including the fact that they can be detected in patient sera, they are stable, and sensitive detection methods are available, such as microarray and polymerase chain reaction."

40. b. Freezing point depression is a colligative property expressed as $T^{\circ}_f - T_f$ and is equal to the colligative molality m_c multiplied by the freezing point depression constant, K_f, which is 1.86 K m_c^{-1}. 0.002 K would actually be the boiling point elevation, $T^{\circ}_b - T_b$, which is equal to the colligative molality m_c multiplied by K_b, which is the boiling point elevation constant (0.513 K m_c^{-1}); 1.15 K is a random number that does not correspond to any constant; and 3.16 K is a value derived by this equation, by using Henry's law constant [for $O_2(g)$ in water at 25 degrees Celsius], which is 790 bar M^{-1}.

41. c. As stated in the text, overexpression of c-Myc, Sox2, Oct4, and Klf4 can reprogram somatic cells into a pluripotent state. C-Myc, Sox2, Oct4, and Klf4 are all transcription factors.

42. d. As described in the text, ESCs and FSCs raise ethical concerns, as well as concerns about tumor formation and immune rejection. Induced pluripotent stem cells could bypass some of these concerns, but they could still carry tumor risk and are difficult to culture. On the other hand, ASCs, such as MSCs and NSCs, have been studied in preclinical and clinical trials for the treatment of neurological disorders.

43. d. Although growth factors are probably required for the maintenance and proliferation of MSCs, it most likely does not have to be a specific subset of them. Similar to other ASCs, MSCs must be adherent, which can be reasoned based on the fact that they serve to replenish cells in environmentally exposed epithelial lining tissue. Additionally, populations of ASCs can be defined by their biomarkers (cell surface markers), which in the case of MSCs are CD73, CD90, and CD105, to name a few, and while MSCs are multipotent and can differentiate into cell types of the resident tissue (bone, cartilage, and adipocytes), they do not necessarily differentiate into neuronal or cardio cells.

44. b. As stated in the passage, MSCs are believed to act via paracrine effects on cells in the surrounding area instead of triggering regeneration of neuronal cells. Paracrine effects include secretion of growth factors, cytokines to modulate the immune system, and anti-apoptotic factors, which have all been reported for MSCs. The passage does not indicate that stem cells secrete pluripotency-inducing factors, such as c-Myc; nor have they been found to have that activity.

45. a. As stated in the passage, *Staphylococcus* is a Gram-positive bacteria and *Staphylococcus aureus* can be distinguished from other *Staphylococcus* species because it is coagulase-positive. *Staphylococcus* bacteria are cocci-shaped and aerobic bacteria (and thus catalase-positive).

46. d. The bacteria in the first image are spherical cells, in the second image are rods, and in the third image are spiral cells. As stated in the passage, *Streptococcus* species are spherical, whereas *E. coli* (as well as *Salmonella bongori*) are rod-shaped. *S. aureus* is sphere-shaped. Both *Treponema pallidum* and *Borrelia burgdorferi* are spiral-shaped.

47. c. Based on the description in the passage, the bacteria is Gram positive. *Bacillus anthracis* is Gram positive, whereas *Salmonella bongori*, *Escherichia coli*, and *Neisseria meningitides* are Gram negative.

48. d. According to Henry's law, the concentration of gas in a liquid is equal to the partial pressure of that gas, in this gas 1 atm, divided by the Henry's law constant kh (atm/M) for that gas. The concentration for He, N_2, O_2, and CO_2 is 0.00037 M, 0.00063 M, 0.0013 M, and 0.034 M, respectively.

49. b. "POMC neurons are anorexigenic because, by activating MC4R, they reduce food intake and increase energy expenditure," so disruption of the POMC gene would be expected to increase fat accumulation. Additionally, the POMC polypeptide is processed into nine proteins including α-MSH, so disruption of the POMC gene would be expected to lead to downregulation of α-MSH, and POMC activates MC4R neurons, so disruption of the POMC gene would be expected to reduce activation of MC4R neurons.

50. c. As stated in the passage, POMC is processed by proteases that cleave in between basic residues. Arg and Lys are basic amino acid residues, Gln is polar, and Asp and Glu are acidic.

51. b. As stated in the passage, binding of leptin to its receptor, Ob-Rb, activates the JAK-STAT pathway. In this canonical signaling pathway, binding (in this case of leptin to two receptor monomers) leads to dimerization of the receptor molecules, followed by phosphorylation of the intracellular regions of the receptor dimer. Then the phosphorylated receptors recruit STAT molecules, which dock, become phosphorylated themselves, dimerize, and then translocate to the nucleus to finally stimulate gene expression.

52. d. The top graph is ghrelin, and the bottom graph is insulin. As stated in the passage, ghrelin acts on a short time scale and is responsible for feelings of sharp hunger. Thus, it peaks right before mealtimes. This pattern is in contrast to insulin and leptin, which repress feelings of hunger and have a longer time scale.

53. b. NK cells are part of the innate immune system, not the adaptive immune system. As can be seen in the graph, NK cells can be activated by interferons (IFNs) and certain cytokines (such as IL-12), the levels of NK cells decline as T-cells are produced, and NK cells help control virus replication in the early days of a viral infection, but they do not eliminate the virus.

54. d. IgM is the first class of immunoglobulin produced after activation of a B cell.

55. d. As stated in the passage, "fatty acid chains with more than 14 carbons are more lipophilic than shorter chains, and unsaturated fatty acids are more likely to undergo lymphatic transport than saturated fatty acids." Phosphatidylcholine has a 16-carbon tail, choline is a head group alcohol with only five carbon atoms, glycerol is a head group alcohol with only three carbon atoms, and palmitic acid is a saturated fatty acid.

56. a. As described in the passage, the inability of a drug to diffuse across the blood vessel endothelium can block its uptake into blood vessels and encourage lymph uptake because lymphatic capillaries are more permeable than blood capillaries. Compounds with larger molecular weight and colloidal materials would be less likely to diffuse easily. Also, as stated in the text, hydrophilic compounds are primarily taken up by blood vessels.

57. b. As stated in the text, CD_{50} is the concentration of drug at which half of the cells die, so the lower the concentration (here in μM) the more toxic the drug. The lowest CD_{50} is that of didanosine-derivative 1.

58. a. Kinesin and dynein are both microtubule motors, and dynein is involved in slow axonal transport. A major difference between kinesin- and dynein-based (and myosin-based) cell motility is that AMP-PNP (adenylyl-imidodiphosphate) dramatically inhibits kinesin activity, but it is only a weak inhibitor of dynein, and dynein is involved in retrograde axonal transport, whereas kinesin is classified as an anterograde axonal transporter.

59. c. The test could not predict AKI on the day of surgery (point 1 = baseline; point 2 = right after surgery; point 3 = 4 hours after surgery) because there was no difference between the patients with AKI (light gray bars) and without AKI (dark gray bars). However, the morning after surgery (point 4), the test is able to predict AKI.

Part 2: Chemical and Physical Foundations of Biological Systems

1. b. This choice is correct. The ideal gas law, $PV = nRT$, is required for this problem to determine the number of moles of air the lungs can hold.

$$n = \frac{PV}{RT} = \frac{(1\ atm)(6.0\ L)}{\left(0.0821\ \frac{L \cdot atm}{mol \cdot K}\right)(310\ K)} = 0.236\ mol \text{ air}$$

Since only 78.1% of the air is nitrogen, this number must be multiplied by 0.781. This gives an answer of 0.184 moles of nitrogen. Finally, this number must be converted to number of molecules using Avogadro's number.

$$0.184\ mol\ N_2 \times \frac{6.022 \times 10^{23}\ \text{molecules}}{1\ mol\ N_2}$$
$$= 1.11 \times 10^{23} \text{ molecules } N_2$$

This calculation shows that choice **a** is too low, choice **d** is too high, and choice **c** would be obtained if one failed to multiply the number of moles by 78.1%.

2. a. $pK_a = -\log(6.28 \times 10^{-5}) = 4.20$
$pH = pK_a + \log \frac{[A^-]}{[HA]} = 4.20 + \log \frac{[0.0800\ M]}{[0.805\ M]}$
$= 3.20$

The Henderson-Hasselbach equation can be used to correctly calculate the pH using the information provided. This calculation shows that the pH in answers **b**, **c**, and **d** are too high.

3. b. $C_2H_5OH(l) + 3O_2(g) \rightarrow 2CO_2(g) + 3H_2O(l)$

5.00 mL ethanol $\times \frac{0.789\,g\,\text{ethanol}}{1\,\text{mL ethanol}} \times \frac{1\,\text{mol ethanol}}{46.1\,g\,\text{ethanol}}$

$\times \frac{3\,\text{mol }H_2O}{1\,\text{mol ethanol}} \times \frac{18\,g\,H_2O}{1\,\text{mol }H_2O} \times \frac{1\,\text{mL }H_2O}{1\,g\,H_2O}$

$= 4.62$ mL water

Percent Yield $= \frac{\text{Actual Yield}}{\text{Theoretical Yield}} \times 100\%$

$= \frac{1.10\,\text{mL water}}{4.52\,\text{mL water}} \times 100\% = 24.3\%$

The calculation above uses the volume, density, and molar mass of ethanol, the correct mole ratio between ethanol and water, and the molar mass and density of water to calculate the theoretical yield of water in the reaction. The percent yield is then calculated by dividing the actual yield by the theoretical yield to find the percent yield for the reaction. Choice **a** would be obtained if the two densities were switched in the calculation; choice **c** would be obtained if the mole ratio for ethanol and carbon dioxide were used instead of the correct mole ratio for ethanol and water; and choice **d** would be obtained if a 1:1 mole ratio were used.

4. c. This choice is correct. Chaotropic agents disrupt hydrogen bond networks by definition, and the structure of urea is particularly suited for this purpose. Within the carbonyl group, the oxygen has a high electronegativity and free electron lone pairs, making it very suitable as a hydrogen bond acceptor. Additionally, the nitrogens are both electronegative and can serve as hydrogen bond acceptors, while the hydrogens on the nitrogens are potential hydrogen bond donors. Molecules like formaldehyde may disturb the covalent or ionic bonds between monomers, but urea is unlikely to do this. Disulfide bond breakage is the result of sulfur reduction. This is commonly caused by such agents as 2-mercaptoethanol and dithiothreitol, but the structure of urea contains no structures likely to accomplish this reaction. Finally, Peptide bond hydrolysis can occur in the presence of water, with 2 to 4 kcal/mol of free energy released per peptide bond. However, this process is extremely slow, and no feature of urea is uniquely suited to speed up this process.

5. d. For all five tested pH values, the denaturation curve shifts to the right as salt concentration increases. A shift to the right indicates that a higher concentration of urea is required to denature the protein, which suggests increased stability. Therefore, increased salt concentration appears to stabilize the protein in this experiment. Increasing salt concentration increases protein stability at all pH values because the elliptical curves consistently shift to the right as salt concentration increases, so there is no significant difference between salt concentration effects at low and high pH.

6. c. The best buffer selection is the one whose pK_a is within 1 pH unit of the desired pH. The only buffer in the provided table that has a pK_a within 1 pH unit of the desired pH in Figure 1, panel c, is HEPES, which has a pK_a of 7.6. None of the pK_a of glycine-HCl, sodium acetate, and ammonium acetate are within 1 pH unit of the desired pH of 7.

7. a. When ΔG is positive, the process under investigation is non-spontaneous and requires external energy to occur. Therefore, an increase in ΔG in this experiment indicates increased resistance to denaturation. As pH increases, the elliptical curves shift to the right, indicating increased resistance to denaturation. This is true for all curves where NaCl is present. Therefore, as pH increases, the unfolding ΔG also increases. Protein stability consistently increases throughout the tested pH range, so the ΔG consistently increases.

8. d. The frequency, inversely proportional to period, measures how quickly the object is oscillating. Velocity is defined as the distance an object travels over a given time frame, acceleration is a measure of the change in velocity over a given time frame, and the period is the amount of time it takes for the spring to complete one oscillation cycle.

9. c. Because potential energy is equal to $\frac{1}{2}kx^2$, changes in m do not affect potential energy, and potential energy stays the same as m increases; additionally, the spring constant does not change for a given spring.

10. a. Potential Energy $= \frac{1}{2}kx^2 = \frac{1}{2}(5.0\,\frac{N}{m})$ $(0.75\,m - 0.5\,m)^2 = 0.63$ J The calculated number and unit are both correct. 1 Joule (J) = 1 Newton (N) × 1 meter (m). Choice **b** would be obtained if one forgot to subtract 0.5 m from the x value, choice **c** if one used the mass instead of the change in spring length, and choice **d** if one incorrectly swapped the k and x values.

11. a. Kinetic energy $= \frac{1}{2}mv^2$, so if kinetic energy is increasing and mass is constant, velocity must also be increasing. Both the kinetic energy and velocity are at their minima when the spring is fully extended and fully compressed, so if kinetic energy is increasing, the box must be moving away from these positions. If the box is moving to the left, its kinetic energy increases as it approaches equilibrium and decreases as it approaches the spring's most compressed state; if the box is moving to the right, its kinetic energy increases as it approaches equilibrium and decreases as it approaches the spring's most extended state.

12. b. The cathode is the negatively charged terminal where the reduction reaction occurs. The anode, by definition, is the positively charged terminal and is the location of the oxidation reaction, and the reduction reaction occurs *only* at the cathode, not at the anode. As a reduction must be occurring, answer **d** cannot be correct.

13. d. The oxidation number of V changes from 4+ to 5+ over the course of the reaction, so V is being oxidized. The oxidation number of H is 1+ in both the reactants and products; Mn changes from 7+ to 4+ over the course of the reaction, so Mn is being reduced; and O is 2– in all species in this reaction.

14. b. The Lewis structure of MnO_4^- is shown below:

There are four possible resonance structures, with the single bond on each of the four oxygens, but for the purposes of VSEPR shapes, these resonance structures are not particularly important. What is important is that there are no lone pairs on the Mn atom that will influence the shape of the molecule. There are four ligands on Mn, and there are no lone pairs on the central atom. Therefore, the shape of the molecule is tetrahedral. There are no lone pairs on Mn that would cause the square planar shape. This shape is usually observed when there are four ligands and two lone pairs on the central atom. Linear configurations most commonly occur in molecules with two ligands on the central atom. And Seesaw configurations commonly occur when there are four ligands and two lone electron pairs on a central atom. Since there are four ligands and no lone pairs on Mn in permanganate, this is not the correct shape.

15. b. We must begin with the provided half-reactions:

$MnO_4^- + 4H^+ + 3e^- \rightarrow MnO_2 + 2H_2O$
E° = 1.68 V
$VO_2^+ + 2H^+ + e^- \rightarrow VO^{2+} + H_2O$ E° = 1.00 V

Based on reduction potentials, the first half-reaction will be the reduction reaction in the spontaneous overall reaction. The equation provided in the question already tells us this. The second half-reaction must therefore be reversed and multiplied by 3; the reduction potential must be reversed to –1.00, but it should *not* be multiplied by 3. The equations can then be added together to get the overall reaction, and the reduction potentials can also be added together to get E° for the cell:

$MnO_4^- + 4H^+ + 3e^- \rightarrow MnO_2 + 2H_2O$
E° = 1.68 V
$3VO^{2+} + 3H_2O \rightarrow VO_2^+ + 6H^+ + 3e^-$
E° = –1.00 V

$MnO_4^- + 3VO^{2+} + H_2O \rightarrow MnO_2 + 6H^+ + 3VO_2^+$ E° = 0.68 V

Finally, the equation $\Delta G° = -nFE°$ is used to calculate $\Delta G°$, keeping in mind that 1 V = 1 J/C:

$\Delta G = -nFE° = -(3 \ mol \ e^-)(96,485 \ \frac{c}{mol})$
$(0.68\frac{J}{C}) = -1.97x10^5 \ J = -197 \ kJ/mol \ MnO_4^-$

Choice **a** would be obtained if one used 1 for *n* rather than 3 during the last step, choice **c** would be obtained if E° for the oxidation half-reaction was multiplied by 3 and then 1, rather than 3, was used for *n* during the last step, and choice **d** would be obtained if E° for the oxidation half-reaction was multiplied by 3 and then everything else was done correctly.

16. c. Plant cells have cellulose cell walls, so *c. reinhardtii* does have a cellulose cell wall. The presence of a cell wall makes lysis more difficult because the purpose of a cell wall is to provide structural stability. There are membrane-bound organelles in *c. reinhardtii* because it is an algal cell and therefore is categorized taxonomically in the Plantae kingdom. However, this feature is not especially relevant to difficulties with cell lysis. Fungal cells have chitin cell walls, but *c. reinhardtii* is a member of the Plantae kingdom. Additionally, Plant cells have nuclei.

17. b. A free asparagine contains two nitrogen atoms: one in its side chain and one in the amine group that forms the peptide bond within a protein. If all ^{14}N atoms are swapped ^{15}N isotopes, the mass of free asparagine should increase by 2 amu.

18. d. As Figure 1 indicates, the R_t value is indeed the fraction of total free amino acids and proteins that are labeled, and the measurement occurs in unlabeled media. The R_t value is a fractional measurement, not an absolute quantity, and the passage explains that the measurement is made *after* transfer to the unlabeled media, and the passage indicates that the R_t measurement is made in unlabeled media.

19. b. SDS is an anionic detergent that linearizes proteins and imparts a negative charge to them, so the SDS-PAGE step is the first step that denatures the proteins of interest. As the cells are still intact and producing protein during this procedure, no protein denaturation has yet occurred. Further protein damage occurs during Trypsin digestion, but denaturation already took place first during SDS-PAGE, and the the SDS-PAGE step already denatured the proteins of interest.

20. c. Oxygen from blood in the capillaries is distributed to all of the body tissues. Oxygen-poor tissues have a high concentration of carbon dioxide, so oxygen diffuses from the blood into the interstitial fluid, but carbon dioxide diffuses from the interstitial fluid into the blood, ammonia is a cellular waste product that moves from the interstitial fluid into the blood, and nitrogen does not significantly diffuse out of the capillaries for distribution to the body tissues.

21. b. The osmotic pressure is less than the hydrostatic pressure at the arteriole end, causing fluid to move from the vessel to the body tissue. Alternatively, the osmotic pressure is greater than the hydrostatic pressure at the venule end, causing fluid, carbon dioxide, and other wastes to be drawn from the body tissue into the capillary vessel. Toward the middle of the capillary bed, the osmotic and hydrostatic blood pressures are equal, resulting in relatively equal fluid flow between the capillary vessel and the body tissue. And the osmotic and hydrostatic blood pressures are opposing forces, so the osmotic pressure itself is not bidirectional on the capillary walls.

22. c. According to the passage, capillaries are narrower than arteries. The continuity equation indicates that when a fluid is forced through a narrow section, it sees an effective velocity increase. Therefore, directing blood to the capillaries should increase the flow rate because the capillaries are thinner than the arteries. Dalton's law describes gas partial pressures and is irrelevant to this and, while the principle in choice **d** is correct, the opposite effect will be observed.

23. b. Blood has a low enough Mach number that it is defined as incompressible in fluid dynamics. Alternatively, blood is non-Newtonian, capillaries are neither long nor straight, and the branching adds an additional layer of complexity, and blood flow is not laminar due to mixing, as the capillary bed is full of branching vessels.

24. b. By definition, convective heat transfer occurs due to bulk motion of fluids. Conductive heat transfer is energy transfer via vibrations at a molecular level through a solid or liquid, answer **c** is not a common term to describe heat transfer, and radiative heat transfer, by definition, is the transfer of energy through electromagnetic waves.

25. b. The area within the cardiac PV loop of each ventricle represents the external work done by that particular ventricle to eject blood, which is a primary function of the ventricle. According to the graph, the area contained within the PV loop for the left ventricle is much greater than the area contained within the PV loop for the right ventricle. Therefore, when looking at the total amount of work done by the ventricles, the left ventricle contraction has contributed more to that total than the right ventricle. It is true that the end-systolic pressure is higher than the end-diastolic pressure, but the same cannot be said about the volumes and, although the circulatory system is generally quite elastic, the data presented here do not necessarily say anything of relevance pertaining to ventricle elasticity.

26. c. The change in length of an object under linear thermal expansion is equal to (initial length, m) × (linear expansion coefficient, m/m°C) × (final temperature – initial temperature). Therefore the change in length of an object under linear thermal expansion is a function of initial length and the magnitude of change in the temperature. The initial length is required, but it is not the only value required, and is only required in conjunction with the final temperature, which means that the magnitude of change in temperature is actually the value of which linear thermal expansion is a function.

27. d. This choice is correct. Curcumin exhibits a strong UV-vis absorbance due to the $\pi \rightarrow \pi^*$ transitions within the conjugated pi bonding system in the molecule. There are two carbonyl groups in curcumin, but they are not linked by an oxygen. Therefore, there is not actually an anhydride group in the molecule. Additionally, the hydroxyl groups alone are not responsible for the UV-vis signal, and spin-spin splitting is relevant in ^{1}H NMR, but it is unrelated to the observed UV-vis signal.

28. b. This Lineweaver-Burk plot represents non-competitive inhibition. The passage states that the K_m stays the same, so the x-intercept should be the same with and without curcumin, as the x-intercept is the negative reciprocal of the K_m. The Vmax decreases when curcumin is added; therefore, the y-intercept of the Lineweaver-Burk plot should increase because it is the reciprocal of the V_{max} value. The plot in choice **a** represents uncompetitive inhibition, while the plot in choice **c** is for competitive inhibition. Finally, although K_m does not change, the V_{max} does decrease.

29. c. Noncompetitive inhibitors change the V_{max} but not the K_m. Competitive inhibitors change the K_m but not the V_{max}, uncompetitive inhibitors change both the K_m and the V_{max}, and irreversible inhibitors bind irreversibly, usually via covalent bonds, to the enzyme's active site, essentially inactivating the enzyme. This is not what these data demonstrate.

30. a. Most fluorescence emissions in proteins are due to excitation of tryptophan residues, with a few emissions due to tyrosine and phenylalanine. These particular amino acids are aromatic and consequently exhibit fluorescence. Tryptophan is a relatively rare amino acid, and its fluorescence is very sensitive. The quenching upon addition of curcumin is likely the result of conformational changes and stacking interactions between aromatic species. Alanine, cysteine, and glutamine residues are all not aromatic or fluorescent.

31. a. This equation correctly relates Gibbs free energy with the dissociation constant K_d. The equation in choice **b** would correctly calculate the k_{cat} value in Michaelis-Menten kinetics, choice **c** is a variation on the equation for calculating the apparent K_m value in the presence of the curcumin inhibitor, and in choice **d** the correct equation has the K_d and ΔG swapped.

32. d. Refracting power (cornea in air) $= \frac{n_{cornea} - n_{air}}{R}$
$= \frac{1.38 - 1.00}{0.0078 \text{ m}} = 48$ diopters

Refracting power (cornea in water)
$= \frac{n_{cornea} - n_{water}}{R} = \frac{1.38 - 1.33}{0.0078 \text{ m}} = 6.4$ diopters

% of refracting power lost
$= \frac{48 \text{ diopters} - 6.4 \text{ diopters}}{48 \text{ diopters}} \times 100\% = 87\%$

Based on the calculation above, this is the percentage of refracting power that is lost when the cornea is submerged in water. Choice **a** is the percentage of refracting power that remains when the cornea is submerged in water, choice **b** is the percentage for the ratio of refractive indices of air to water, and choice **c** is the opposite percentage for the ratio of refractive indices of air to water.

33. d. The image equation can be used to solve for the effective focal length:
$\frac{1}{f} = \frac{1}{d_0} + \frac{1}{d_i} = \frac{1}{1,000 \text{ mm}} + \frac{1}{17.0 \text{ mm}} = 0.0598$
$f = 16.7$ mm

Based on the calculation above, this is the correct effective focal length for the average eye for an object positioned 1 meter away. The inverse of choice **a** is true, while choice **b** is one decimal place off from the inverse value in choice **a**, and choice **c** is one decimal place off from the correct answer in choice **d**.

34. c. This is the correct angle of refraction, based on the following calculation, which uses Snell's law:
$\theta 2 = \sin^{-1}\left(\frac{n_1 \sin\theta_1}{n_2}\right) = \sin^{-1}\left(\frac{1.00 \sin(80.0°)}{1.38}\right)$
$= 45.5°$

Choice **a** is the complementary angle to the incident angle, choice **b** is the complementary angle to the correct answer, and choice **d** is the angle of incidence.

35. b. If the eye is too long, the light rays are apt to focus before reaching the retina, causing myopia. Other causes include altered curvature of the lens and cornea. Insufficient refractive power would cause farsightedness, the refractive index would not fluctuate significantly to cause myopia, and, as myopia is entirely the result of what is happening before any light rays hit the retina, defects in the retina itself do not cause myopia.

36. c. The electric field of circularly polarized light moves around an axis in the direction of propagation at a constant angular velocity. Choice **a** is true of linearly polarized light, not circularly polarized light. Choice **b** is mostly true, except for the fact that angular velocity remains constant with circularly polarized light, as is choice **d**, except for the fact that angular velocity remains constant with circularly polarized light.

37. b. The hydroxide from a base, like NaOH or KaOH, attacks the carbonyl of the ester, forming a carboxylic acid. Triglycerides are esters by definition, and saponification only occurs under basic conditions.

38. c. γ decay occurs when a nucleus in an excited energy state emits a gamma ray, transitioning it to a lower energy state but leaving the atomic number unchanged. α decay decreases the atomic number by 2, β decay decreases (or increases, for β^+ decay) the atomic number by 1, and the atomic number decreases by 1 in electron capture.

39. b. The general trend in ionic radii for cations, particular for the alkali and alkaline earth metals, is that ions become larger as you move to the left and down on the periodic table. Moving down the periodic table increases the number of energy levels, while moving left decreases effective nuclear charge. Patterns are inconsistent within the transition metals, but all transition metals in the top rows are smaller than the alkali and alkaline earth metals in the same row, so the nickel and zinc ions are smaller than the calcium ion.

40. b. This is the structure of L-ornithine. The passage states that the arginase reaction involves the hydrolysis of arginine, with urea and L-ornithine as the products. The chemical formula for urea is provided. Given the definition of a hydrolysis by nucleophilic water, the two reactants and one product, and the UV-vis absorbance at 515 nm (indicating the presence of an amine group), the structure of L-ornithine can therefore be elucidated. Choice **a** is the structure of L-canavanine. This structure is very similar to arginine, except there is an extra oxygen inserted, choice **c** is the structure of L-lysine, and choice **d** is the structure of L-citrulline.

41. d. The passage states that *H. pylori* prefers cobalt at pH 6. RocF from *B. anthracis* prefers nickel at pH 9 (followed by Mn^{2+} and Co^{2+}), based on the data in Figure 1. Therefore, *B. anthracis* RocF has a different metal preference and a different optimal pH relative to the arginase from *H. pylori*.

42. c. The order of metal preference at pH 6.3 is $Ni^{2+} > Mn^{2+} > Co^{2+}$, while at pH 9, the order of metal preference is $Ni^{2+} > Co^{2+} > Mn^{2+}$. The data in Figure 1 only reflect the rate of arginase reaction. No conclusions can be drawn about metal binding affinities from these data, Figure 1 is not an assay that directly measures viable cell growth, and the levels of L-ornithine are measured after 24 hours, so the overall production of product is measured, not the rate of reaction.

43. a. The pK_a for the side group of the aspartate residues is around 2.4, so both should be negatively charged at pH 6. Histidine has a pK_a around 6, so it should not be charged above pH 6. Both alanine and glycine will not be charged. Therefore, most of the residues should be uncharged at the provided pH values. Histidine can be positively charged, and it can interact with the metal through its pi bonds. Histidine has pK_a around 6, but it should not be charged above pH 6. Of the five, only histidine is aromatic, and only alanine and glycine are hydrophobic.

44. b. Figure 1 shows that nickel is highly preferred, but in vivo, its presence does not result in high arginase activity, which means that RocF in vivo only seems to have access to manganese, even though it is not the preferred metal. Figure 2 shows measurements of arginase activity from harvested cells, not actual cell growth. The cells still grew even though the cobalt and nickel trials showed no significant arginase activity. The passage even states directly that cell growth occurred by noting that cells were harvested and assayed for the viable cell arginase assay. Significant arginase activity is observed in vivo in *B. anthracis* in the presence of manganese, and Figures 1 and 2 do not measure reaction rate, so the conclusion in choice **d** is not supported by any of the data collected.

45. b. If the CRR' carbon bonded with the carbon of the protonated formaldehyde, a less stable primary carbocation would form. The electronegativity difference actually goes the other direction than indicated in choice **a**, giving the CH_2 carbon slightly *more* electron pull than the CRR' carbon since C has a higher electronegativity than H, and Hückel's rule helps to determine if a planar ring molecule is aromatic. It is not relevant to this reaction in any way. Finally, it is actually more sterically favorable for the CRR' carbon to bond with the carbon on the protonated formaldehyde, because it would keep the larger R and R' groups farther away from the rest of the molecule.

46. a. An elimination reaction removes two substituents from a molecule to form a double bond. A hydrolysis reaction involves the breaking of a bond in a molecule using water, while a tautomerization reaction is essentially a conversion to an isomer that often results in the formal migration of a hydrogen atom, and a nucleophilic substitution reaction involves the selective attack by an electron nucleophile to replace a leaving group.

47. b. Because a dioxane and 1,3-diol form, the reaction conditions must include a protic acid, a temperature lower than 70°C, and an excess of formaldehyde. $(CH_3)_2CO$ is not a protic acid, the temperature is over 70°C, and the alkene is in excess.

48. d. Answer **a** does not correctly identify the four-carbon chain as the longest chain of carbons upon which to base the name, choice **b** does not match the structure at all, and in choice **c** the carbons in the four-carbon chain have been numbered backwards. C1 should be the carbon at the end of the chain with the hydroxyl group.

$$
\begin{array}{c}
OH \\
| \\
H-C-H \\
| \\
H-C-H \\
| \\
H_3C-C-OH \\
| \\
CH_3
\end{array}
$$

The carbons are numbered correctly, and all side groups are identified correctly.

49. c. There are two carbons on each oxygen, and there are also two lone pairs of electrons, each of which occupies a hybrid orbital, and choice **d** is not a relevant type of hybridization here.

50. c. LSD has two chiral centers and therefore $2^2 (4)$ unique stereoisomers.

51. b. The other two nitrogens are much less basic due to resonance effects and aromaticity. The lone pair in choice **a** is in resonance with the C=O carbonyl group, which makes the nitrogen significantly less basic, while the lone pair on the nitrogen in choice **c** is a part of the aromatic ring system, per Hückel's rule. This effectively makes this nitrogen also much less basic. Because resonance effects and aromaticity significantly decrease the basicity of nitrogen 1 and nitrogen 3, nitrogen 2 is clearly the most basic of the three.

52. a. The carboxamide group is electron withdrawing, largely due to its carbonyl group, which consequently makes the C-8 proton more labile. Choice **b** is actually the reason why the C-5 proton is labile, although the C-8 proton is significantly *more* labile than the C-5 proton, steric stress here is not a reason to explain why the C-8 proton is labile, and although LSD is largely planar, the planarity does not contribute to the lability of the C-8 proton.

53. c. This is the IR spectrum for piperidine. There is a weak band at 3,300 (2° amine stretching), 1,600 (2° amine bending), 3,000 (alkane stretching), and 1,450 (alkane bending). Choice **a** is not the IR spectrum for acetamide because there are no bands around 1,720 (C=O stretching). There is also not a double band around 3,400–3,500 (1° amine). Choice **b** cannot be correct because there are no sharp bands around 2,240–2,260 for the cyanide group, and choice **d** is not the IR spectrum for benzoic acid. There are no bands around 1,705–1,720 (C=O stretching) or benzene ring bands.

54. c. In a gas reaction like this, decreasing the pressure will shift the reaction in the direction that produces more moles of gas. Therefore, decreasing the pressure will shift the equilibrium to the left. Adding a catalyst has no effect on equilibrium, adding O_2 will shift the equilibrium to the right, and decreasing the temperature favors the exothermic reaction, which shifts the equilibrium to the right.

55. b. The graph shows that lysine, like arginine, is positively charged in an amino group on the end of a chain. The only feature that arginine has that all of the other tested residue 188 residues lack is the ability to form a bidentate H-bond, which is likely essential for substrate binding since the substrate sucrose has several hydroxyl groups. The polarity of residue 188 is important because it exists in the transmembrane region, as sucrose must be transported through the hydrophobic interior of the lipid bilayer, but both H and K are positively charged at pH 4.0 and did not result in a functional protein. The results obtained say nothing about hydrophobic residues because none were tested here, but because residue 188 is located in the transmembrane region of OsSUT1, residue 188 likely needs to be hydrophilic for sucrose transport through the hydrophobic interior of the lipid bilayer. And every residue tested in place of R188 was smaller in size and still did not allow for a functional protein.

56. d.

$$H_2S + NO_3^- \rightarrow S_8 + NO$$

$$H_2S \rightarrow S_8 \qquad\qquad NO_3^- \rightarrow NO$$

$$8H_2S \rightarrow S_8 \qquad\qquad NO_3^- \rightarrow NO$$

$$NO_3^- \rightarrow NO + 2H_2O$$

$$8H_2S \rightarrow S_8 + 16H^+ \qquad NO_3^- \rightarrow + 4H^+ \rightarrow NO + 2H_2O$$

$$8H_2S \rightarrow S_8 + 16H^+ + 16e^- \qquad NO_3^- + 4H^+ + 3e^- \rightarrow NO + 2H_2O$$

$$\times 3 \qquad\qquad\qquad \times 16$$

$$24H_2S \rightarrow 3S_8 + 48H^+ + 48e^- \qquad 16NO_3^- + 64H^+ + 48e^- \rightarrow 16NO + 32H_2O$$

$$\overline{\qquad\qquad\qquad\qquad\qquad\qquad\qquad\qquad\qquad\qquad\qquad\qquad\qquad}$$

$$24H_2S + 16NO_3^- + 64H^+ + 48e^- \rightarrow 3S_8 + 48H^+ + 48e^- + 16NO + 32H_2O$$

$$24H_2S + 16NO_3^- + 16H^+ \rightarrow 3S_8 + 16NO + 32H_2O$$

The balanced equation above shows that the coefficient for H_2S is 24.

57. d. The data indicate that the reaction is zero-order in [A] and second-order in [B]. That means that the rate law is $k[B]^2$, and the linear plot should be $[B]^{-1}$ vs. t to determine slope k.

58. c. The fractional distillation setup requires a heat source and condenser. The liquid with the lower boiling point evaporates first and is condensed for collection, and so on, allowing for liquid separation. Fractional distillation separates liquids based on their boiling points and choice **d** actually describes an organic extraction.

59. a. The product is neutral overall, but internally it includes a positive and negative charge. Therefore, the product is one zwitterionic compound.

$$CH_3OH \; + \; BF_3 \; \rightleftharpoons \; CH_3 \overset{\overset{\displaystyle H}{|}}{\underset{\oplus}{O}} \overset{\ominus}{-} BF_3$$

Part 3: Psychological, Social, and Biological Foundations of Behavior

1. d. Around eighth or ninth grade, students are transitioning to formal operational thought, which includes both propositional logic and combinatorial reasoning. This study is about individual cognition; Erikson's work dealt with how individuals relate to the social world. And according to Freud's theory, child development occurs in a series of stages focused on different pleasure areas of the body. During each stage, the child encounters conflicts that play a major role in the course of development. Finally, Maslow focused on a hierarchy of needs. This study was not needs based.

2. a. Deductive logic is a logical process in which a conclusion is based on the concordance of multiple premises that are generally assumed to be true. Children in the concrete operational stage have problems with this concept. Perspective taking is defined as viewing the world from something other than one's habitual vantage point. Children have trouble with this in the preoperational stage of development. Inductive logic involves going from a specific experience to a general principle. Children in the concrete operational stage are fairly adept at this. And conservation refers to a logical thinking ability that is present in the preoperational stage of development.

3. b. The majority of students moved from the concrete to operational levels. There was no difference between the two treatment groups, relaxation was not studied in this study, and the difference between combinatorial reasoning and propositional logic was not tested in this study.

4. c. Descriptive statistics are used to describe the basic features of the data in a study. They provide simple summaries about the sample and the measures. Inferential statistics reach conclusions that extend beyond the immediate data alone. Inferential statistics try to infer from the sample data what the population might think. Estimates fall under inferential statistics. Estimations are made about a population based on sample data. And modeling falls under inferential statistics and makes a set of assumptions concerning the generation of the observed data and similar data from a larger population.

5. d. During the transition to formal operational thought, children are also experiencing puberty. Physiologically, the frontal lobe of the brain begins more complex development that can continue all the way until early adulthood. The limbic system, which governs emotion, is not altered, the brain structure changes, but the structure is not located in the memory storage area, and the brain structures DO change as the individual moves from one stage to another.

6. b. Maslow places physiological and safety needs near the bottom of his hierarchy of learning. Children who go to school hungry or in fear from violence in their neighborhoods will not be able to concentrate as well as their more affluent peers who are well fed and relatively safe. Although it is possible that there is a correlation between living in poverty and violent crime, choice **a** is not based on a child's failure to meet lower-level needs as suggested by Maslow's hierarchy. Choice **c** is based on Piagetian theory and choice **d** is based on Vygotsky's theory, not Maslow's hierarchy of needs.

7. a. The sense of having always known someone whom we just met is a sign of attachment, although it is sometimes absent in the romantic love sequence. This sense is a sign of attachment, not attraction. Love can occur within the romantic love sequence, but it is not always a part of it, and lust is the sexual component of love and is not described in this question.

8. d. Lateralization of cortical functions allows for parallel processing. Both the right and left brain are involved in parallel processing, and conus medullaris is the tapered end of the inferior end of the spinal cord.

9. d. Associative learning is related to spatial cognition and cognitive mapping. Reinforcement is a type of operant conditioning, avoidance learning is a type of operant conditioning, and spontaneous recovery occurs with classical conditioning.

10. b. Parents do use strategies to help their children overcome social thinking difficulties. Many people who have social thinking difficulties do not have a diagnosis, research does in fact support the hypothesis that teaching methodologies help children overcome social thinking difficulties, and social learning begins during infancy.

11. c. Research has shown that interventions are effective on individuals who have scored near average to very high on intelligence measures. Social thinking is not a natural process for a large number of people, many people with social thinking difficulties have high IQs, and while there are few interventions available, they are effective with individuals who do NOT have a diagnosis.

12. b. The dependent variable does relate directly to the outcome of the study. While the control group is used in the study, it does not relate directly to the outcome. The experimental group is used to compare the outcome to the control group; it is part of the design and is not used as the outcome variable. The independent variable sets up the experimental and non-experimental structure of the study; it does not relate directly to the outcome of the experiment.

13. d. Social thinking is an intuitive process, so it is taken for granted. Social thinking is not related to IQ, people with high-functioning social thinking do learn it from the environment, but those with low-functioning social thinking do not learn it naturally from the environment, and many people with social thinking disorders do NOT have a diagnosis.

14. a. Both parents and professional practitioners have found her treatment programs useful.

15. b. Synaptic vesicles are clustered beneath the membrane in the axon terminal located at the presynaptic side of the synapse. They contain neurotransmitters, which are released through the presynaptic terminal and travel to a destination neuron, binding to the postsynaptic axon terminal. The axon is a projection off of the neuron and is responsible for conducting electrical impulses away from the neuron's cell body. Dendrites are the threadlike extensions of the cytoplasm of a neuron. They are responsible for sending action potentials to the cell body; they do not store neurotransmitters. And there is no cytoplasmic connection between two neurons.

16. c. Cocaine acts by blocking the removal of dopamine from the synapse, which results in the accumulation of an abnormal amplified signal to the dopamine receptors. Serotonin is typically related to major depression, not cocaine use, while glutamate is related to schizophrenia and is not associated with cocaine use, and norepinephrine is not associated with cocaine use.

17. a. Mental health workers have a high incidence of vicarious emotional trauma. People who treat patients with bipolar disorder and schizophrenia tend to have vicarious emotional trauma, not the patients themselves, and people who observe and interact with the individuals with alcoholism often have vicarious emotional trauma.

18. d. Mirror neurons are neurons that fire both when an animal acts and when the animal observes the same action performed by another. The neuron "mirrors" the behavior of the other, as though the observer were acting itself. This is important in self-regulation, which is implicated in autism and schizophrenia. Mirror neuron dysfunction is not typically found in patients with bipolar disorder or major depression, PTSD or eating disorders, or obsessive-compulsive disorder or antisocial personality disorder.

19. c. An imbalance in neurotransmitters may contribute to anxiety disorders. The neurotransmitters targeted in anxiety disorders are gamma-aminobutyric acid (GABA), serotonin, dopamine, and epinephrine. Problems with axons do not cause mental disorders, while the neuron does relate to neurotransmitters, the neuron itself is not the cause, and substance abuse can cause problems with neurotransmitters.

20. a. The teachers who did NOT receive the intervention are known as the control group. The teachers who DID receive the intervention are known as the experimental group, the dependent variable is the variable that changes or does not change as a result of the study, and the independent variable in this study is whether or not the teachers received the intervention.

21. d. One of the factors contributing to the lack of success in the program in THIS study was teachers' desire to conform to their community. The teachers thought that one of the reasons they did NOT work was lack of administrative support, but this is not a reasonable conclusion from THIS study. The results of this study lend support to the conclusion that bullying can be reduced, but the study in and of itself was not sufficient to make this claim. And choice **c** is a future hypothesis that is a logical follow-up to this study but not a reasonable conclusion of THIS study.

22. b. The treatment in the study caused the teachers to reexamine their own views, and this resulted in cognitive dissonance. Adaptation would include the actual restructuring resulting from the cognitive dissonance caused in the study. While cultural conformity was an important variable influencing the results, the teachers' personal experiences in this study caused cognitive dissonance, not conformity. And the independent variable was whether the teachers received the intervention, not what resulted from the intervention.

23. a. Gender is a socially constructed variable. Sex is a biological variable, age is a variable dependent on when the students are born, and the treatment length is a variable in the experimental design—none are socially constructed.

24. a. The hidden curriculum shows up in this study as educational institutions reinforce a societal view that schools should prepare students for the real world, in this case discrimination and bullying due to gender identification. Choice **b** identifies an aspect of experimental design, not the hidden curriculum, choice **c** is consistent with the visible curriculum, that we teach students to be fair to everyone, regardless of gender identification, and choice **d** is an example of blame, not the hidden curriculum.

25. b. Cultural assimilation occurs when new members of a culture take actions to fit into the existing culture to facilitate their becoming part of the new culture. Accommodation is the opposite of the correct answer, which is assimilation. Accommodation occurs when the existing members of the culture change to fit the cultural mores of the new culture, thus changing the existing culture. Functionalism pertains to the different parts of a culture working together as a system. This scenario refers to a much more specific situation. And stratification is what divides cultures into individual, usually ranked, classes. In this case, had one of the two cultures been relegated to a position above or below the other, it would have been stratification.

26. a. Animals adapt to their environment but do not use adaptation as a signal to communicate with other animals. Apes, dogs, and ravens, in particular, use gaze following as a form of communication and signaling. Fish, for example, can give off a faint electromagnetic field that plays a part in predator-prey relationships. And olfaction is one of the oldest methods of communication but is difficult to study because of intervening variables.

27. d. Drive reduction theory says that humans are motivated to reduce the state of tension caused when certain biological needs are not satisfied. Developed by Clark Hull in 1943, it was the first theory of motivation. Incentive theory states that motivations are driven by the desire for external rewards, but this was not the first theory of motivation. Arousal theory maintains our motivations are based upon the notion of keeping an arousal at an equilibrium. This was not the first theory of motivation. An example of humanistic theory is Maslow's hierarchy of needs, and this was not the first theory of motivation.

28. d. Stress that is considered good becomes distressing at the point of fatigue. Ill health effects occur after stress has become distressing for a long period of time, good stress can occur after the comfort zone is achieved, and performance slightly increases even when stress becomes distressful.

29. b. An experimental design is one in which a controlled experimental factor is subjected to special treatment for purposes of comparison, with a factor kept constant. A case study is an in-depth study of a particular research problem, usually with a single individual or topic. Cross-sectional research designs have three distinctive features: no time dimension, a reliance on existing differences rather than change following intervention, and groups that are selected based on existing differences. The cross-sectional design can only measure differences between or from among a variety of people or subjects. And descriptive research designs provide answers to the questions of who, what, when, where, and how associated with a particular research problem.

30. b. The graph is a common example of research that came out of the James-Lange theory. Cannon-Bard worked to refute the James-Lange theory, Piaget and Maslow did not do work in this area, and Schachter-Singer theory came much later than James-Lange.

31. d. Filling out and signing the IRB form is strict protocol for studies with human subjects. The IRB form is intended to protect the subjects and must be turned in; if it is turned in 2 weeks late, damage could already have occurred to the subject; and as it is meant to protect the participants, the form must be turned in before the start of the study.

32. c. This is an example of James-Lange theory, which is still accepted today. Choice **a** is an example of Schachter-Singer theory, choice **b** is an example of Cannon-Bard theory, and choice **d** is the reverse of James-Lange theory.

33. a. Peer pressure and the activities that go with it, like bullying and gossip, can cause depression in teens. Exercise can help with the symptoms of depression, while cutting and promiscuity are associated with depression, not causes of it, and cutting back on social activity is a sign that a teen is already depressed.

34. b. School is a place where a lot of stressors take place, and it is where teens spend a large amount of time. Although mass media can be a stressor, the school setting is more likely to lead to teen depression. Church is a generally positive agent of socialization, and most teens do not work. Those that do would spend much less time there than at school.

35. a. Music is a classic example of symbolic interactionism. It is central to many teens' lives, and the type of music they listen to can influence their identity formation. Through music, they attach meanings to their relationships with the world and themselves. The majority of teens do not emulate their favorite movie and television stars, and even those who do tend to maintain the same gender identity. Additionally, mass media tends to negatively affect teens' self-efficacy (having to be thin, popular, etc.), and class identity is not likely to be affected by mass media.

36. d. A positive family life is most likely to prevent teen depression. Although church may help teens avoids depression, it is not the support system that is most likely to prevent it. Although exercise is positive, physical education class can be the location of bullying and body image problems, and, relatedly, school is the source of many of the stressors affecting teens and is more likely to cause depression than to help prevent it.

37. c. Mass media can make teens feel negative about their appearance and thus can significantly lower their self-efficacy. Family life can be a major stressor in teens' lives, but other stressors affect self-efficacy more, while teens' favorite music tends to make them happier and have higher self-efficacy in most cases, and the workplace can be a positive part of a teen's life and is much less likely than the other choices to lower self-efficacy.

38. a. The child has the concrete knowledge that A (lightning) causes B (thunder) but does not understand the abstract reasoning of *how* A causes B. While the child understands that A causes B, in order to be formal operational, he or she must be able to understand the abstract concept of how lightning's static electricity interacts with air to cause thunder. Similarly, the preoperational child would be able to identify lightning and thunder separately but would not be able to understand the concept of causation between the two, and the sensory-motor child would see lightning and perhaps react, and would hear thunder and perhaps react, but would have no concrete knowledge of either of the two entities.

39. c. Ethnocentrism is the evaluation of other cultures according to preconceptions originating in the standards and customs of one's own culture. Cultural relativism is the principle of regarding the beliefs, values, and practices of a culture from the viewpoint of that culture itself. Therefore, both can be found in individuals and specific nations.

40. d. Group polarization refers to the tendency for groups to make decisions that are more extreme than the initial inclination of its members. Deindividuation is losing self-awareness in a group, deviance is departure from usual or accepted standards, and groupthink is when the desire for harmony or conformity in the group results in an irrational or dysfunctional decision-making outcome.

41. a. Persuasion is a major component of the elaboration likelihood model, but not a major component of social cognitive theory, enculturation theory, or the observational learning model.

42. d. Impression management is a conscious or subconscious process in which people attempt to influence other people's perceptions of a person, object, or event; they do so by regulating and controlling information in social interaction. They could be trying to influence perceptions about themselves or others. Although gender plays a role in the interviewing process, it is not what she is practicing in this scenario; speech is part of the scenario; and although choice **c** includes a social interaction, it is not the main theory operating here.

43. b. Gentrification is the process of renewal and rebuilding accompanying the influx of middle-class or affluent people into deteriorating areas that often displaces poorer residents. Urban blight is the process whereby a previously functioning city, or part of a city, falls into disrepair, often due to environmental factors. Meritocracy is the process in which people's progress is based on ability and talent rather than on class privilege or wealth and intergenerational mobility refers to changes in social status between different generations within the same family. And even though gentrification may integrate neighborhoods, the original residents continue to be marginalized, so social stratification remains in place.

44. a. Good healthcare tends to be lacking in these neighborhoods before gentrification occurs. Housing values are likely to increase with gentrification, the question describes local inequalities, not global, and people moving into the neighborhoods would likely bring an increase in wealth, so poverty is not something they would experience.

45. c. When a neighborhood becomes more popular, residents will need easier ways to travel to and from their home neighborhood to work and other parts of the city. Accessibility of a neighborhood makes it a more desirable place to live. While residents may push for more parks, it is not something that will "have to be improved" in the gentrified neighborhood. The type and variety of restaurants in a neighborhood often changes because of gentrification, but it is not a requirement to create a gentrified neighborhood, and the pace of change in the neighborhood happens on its own and does not need to be improved.

46. d. Students from the existing neighborhood may be displaced due to socioeconomic reasons—their parents might not be able to afford to live in the newly gentrified neighborhood. All children will experience hidden curriculum within the education system, in-group bias refers to a pattern of favoring members of one's in-group over out-group members—both groups of students are likely to experience bias—and a meritocracy is a social system in which people's success in life depends primarily on their talents, abilities, and effort, so both groups of students will experience this through the grading structures used in the education system.

47. b. Poor families are unlikely to be able to afford to live in areas with rising property values and increasing rents. Assimilation is less likely to occur. Existing families are likely to move out, and the new families will determine the new culture of the neighborhood. Additionally, violence in families will not necessarily change due to gentrification, and culture lag has to do with changes due to technology, not gentrification.

48. a. A correlation is a statistical measure that indicates the extent to which two or more variables fluctuate together. A correlational relationship does not mean it is causal. There would need to be evidence that high health beliefs cause high self-concepts. Scores on one measurement cannot predict scores on the other, and if there were variability when examining the measures, a positive relationship would not have been found.

49. c. Locus of control in psychology refers to the extent to which individuals believe they can control events affecting them. It is based on two conditions. A person with an internal locus of control believes that she has control over her life—that life is not based on chance. A person with an external locus of control believes she is powerless and that events that occur and happen to her are based on factors from the environment or due completely to chance. Choice **a** is the definition of the construct health beliefs as used in the study, choice **b** a definition of self-concept, and choice **d** the definition of self-esteem.

50. d. The dependent variable is the outcome of the experiment that determines whether the hypothesis was supported. The control group is the group that does not receive the treatment, the treatment group is the group that does receive the treatment, and the training the experimental group received is the independent variable.

51. b. Obedience is compliance with an order, request, or law or submission to another's authority. The key aspect of obedience is that just because you have changed in some way does not mean that you agree with the change. The nurse followed orders because they came from a perceived authority figure. Peer pressure is influence from members of one's peer group. A doctor would be in a position of authority, not a peer; the bystander effect occurs when individuals do not offer any means of help to a victim when other people are also present; and social loafing is the phenomenon of people exerting less effort to achieve a goal when they work in a group than when they work alone.

52. b. The passage explains signal detection theory, a means to quantify the ability to discern between information-bearing patterns and random patterns that distract from the information. The random patterns are called noise and involve random activity of the detection machine and of the nervous system of the operator. Sensory adaptation is a change over time in the responsiveness of the sensory system to a constant stimulus, the somatosensory system relates to a sensation (such as pressure, pain, or warmth) that can occur anywhere in the body, and Weber's law quantifies the perception of change in a given stimulus. It states that the change in a stimulus that will be just noticeable is a constant ratio of the original stimulus.

53. a. The doctor's neural activity is an example of internal noise. In signal detection theory, internal noise refers to the fact that neural response will be different even if the external stimulus presented is the same every time. In the example above, the CT of the lung is the same in each instance, but the neural activity of the doctor will be different with each viewing. External noise is external to the doctor and may be, for example, a smudge on the film; internal response is the decision the doctor makes in her brain after the internal and external noise have been taken into account; and uncertainty pertains to the overall theory of signal detection, not a specific part of it.

54. a. Psychophysics is the branch of psychology that deals with the relationships between physical stimuli and mental phenomena. Gestalt psychology has to do with the sum being greater than the parts, neuroscience studies the structure or function of the nervous system and brain, and cognitive psychology is the study of how we think, remember, decide, and perceive.

55. c. In an experimental design, the control group and experimental group are the same, except the experimental group is the one in which some type of manipulation has been enacted that was not done to the control group. Since there are two groups and the attending physicians are the control group, the first-year residents are the experimental group. The dependent variable is the outcome of the decisions the doctors make about the images, the independent variable is the set of images used in the study, and there is no treatment group in this study.

56. d. Neuroscience studies the function of the brain, which is clearly depicted in this quote. Choice **a** deals more with cognitive science than neuroscience, uncertainty is inherent in signal detection theory, not neuroscience, as presented in this passage, and choice **c** is an example of external noise.

57. c. When a condition that the learner does not like is removed to reinforce a desired behavior, it is negative reinforcement. In this case, solitary confinement is removed to reinforce the good behavior exhibited by the prisoner. Extinction removes a behavior entirely through classical conditioning. There is no indication the behavior will not return; nor is classical conditioning used. Classical conditioning is an example of negative reinforcement, which is a type of operant conditioning, not classical conditioning, and positive reinforcement would be if the prisoner was given something he or she wanted, such as a particular book to read, to reinforce positive behavior.

58. b. All of the symptoms in the question are signs of elder abuse. People with MS will typically show bruises if they're walking and their coordination is affected, but social withdrawal and arguments with the caregiver are not typical symptoms of the disease.

59. c. Labeling theory is how self-identification and behavior of individuals may be determined or influenced by the terms, or "labels," used to describe them. Self-fulfilling prophecy, as described in the question, would fall under this theory. Differential association theory is the theory that through interaction with others, individuals learn the values, attitudes, techniques, and motives for criminal behavior. Strain theory states that social structures within society may pressure citizens to commit crimes. And behaviorism takes the view that learning occurs through rote memorization and is not a key component of criminology.

Part 4: Critical Analysis and Reasoning Skills

1. c. Goldman argues throughout the passage that when art deals with pressing social issues, it can inspire change more effectively than political speech. In the last paragraph, she discusses how American drama fails to inspire social significance. Goldman might argue that European drama is therefore superior, but the larger point of the passage is that American drama has not yet realized its potential for social change. Goldman might agree with the statement in choice **b**, but rather than saying political speakers need to get their message out through creative work, the main point of her passage is the opposite—that creative work has the power to inspire political/social change. Finally, Goldman mentions art for art's sake in the opening of the passage but moves on from there to discuss art as a "mirror to life."

2. a. Historically, political speakers would give impromptu speeches on social issues on the street, often standing on a shipping crate as their "stage." The term has come to take on a metaphorical meaning. The phrase has no implication regarding the height of the orator, and while soapbox orators may be eloquent, the term addresses the political or social nature of their speech rather than the purity of their language—nor does it have anything to do with actual soap or cleanliness.

3. c. Goldman mentions that American drama has been used for amusement only and that Americans have not had access to European drama in print. The implication is that European drama contains social ideas or political messages that the average American theatergoer has yet to experience. While the statement in choice **a** is true and something the reader can infer, it is not something Goldman could imply, since she would have had no knowledge of the Internet. Additionally, Goldman discusses the availability of theater in America and does not consider a theatergoer's ability to travel; therefore, choice **b** does not imply that it would never happen—and Goldman says that plays have not been available in print, so whether or not the average American would like to read a European play is irrelevant.

4. b. In the context of the passage, Goldman discusses the effectiveness of the language of art and its ability to embrace the "entire gamut of human emotions," which is more moving than the examples of "stereotyped phrases" used by the "average radical." Goldman advocates the use of art as a means of advocating social ideals, but she provides these examples of language as overused, ineffective political speech, and while she uses the term "symbols of revolt," these are not Strindberg's symbols; rather, they are examples of the speech of radicals and conservatives. Finally, Goldman compares radicals to the "man devoid of all ideas": they are both strapped to their limited terminology. The phrases provided aren't actually devoid of all ideas, but Goldman suggests they are as trite as if they were.

5. a. Whistler is advocating the notion of "art for art's sake." Goldman says this type of art "presupposes an attitude of aloofness on the part of the artist" and distinguishes modern art as one that speaks in a "language embracing the entire gamut of human emotions." Goldman dismisses this notion of art. Elsewhere, Goldman does not really discuss artist intention and therefore would not likely advocate its irrelevance and, while the passage focuses on dramatic art, Goldman makes statements about art in general, even saying "those who wield the pen or brush" to indicate that social implications of art apply to both drama and painting. Additionally, the statement in choice **d** is not really a response to Whistler's claim about art, and although Goldman's comments feature a discussion of radical and conservative politicians, she does not criticize their ideals as "clap-trap" but rather criticizes the effectiveness of their methods for expressing their ideas.

6. d. Goldman mentions "those who wield the brush or pen" (i.e., the writer or painter) as being overlooked by politicians, when in fact powerful social messages may be communicated through art. Goldman specifically mentions Walt Whitman as one of the writers whose work mirrors the social revolt of his time, but the bumper sticker takes a tiny phrase of his larger work and reduces it to a slogan. While it contains his words, the bumper sticker is not really an example of Whitman's art. An advertisement, whether containing dramatic actors or not, is closer to the propagandist's speech mentioned by Goldman than the "creative genius, imbued with the spirit of sincerity and truth." Finally, Goldman quotes Strindberg, who equates the dramatist with a "lay preacher," but dismisses the religious nature of Strindberg's metaphor. Martin Luther King Jr. was a preacher whose orations moved many for social change, but he was not known as an artist. Goldman focuses on the power of art for social change.

7. b. Anderson's overall point is that Stein is doing something important with words, elevating plain words, "recasting" everyday words into poetry. The "money saving words" that follow this quote may mislead a reader to agree with choice **a**, but the language is metaphorical—so it does not mean she was literally a housekeeper or had to scrimp and save but instead says something of the language she used in her poetry. Anderson is using metaphorical language to describe Stein's poetry, which uses words that would not traditionally be considered poetic. Further, Anderson does not indicate that Stein has a social message in her poetry but considers the words she uses as "neglected citizens"; Stein is not literally speaking about neglected citizens.

8. b. Anderson praises Stein's work in a defensive mode, suggesting that the "loud guffaws" are those of Stein's critics, indicating also his wish that at least writers would attempt to understand her work. He clearly praises Stein and says the loud guffaws "do not irritate me"—if the guffaws indicated delight, he would not mention irritation—and implies that the guffaws at her work are more mocking than genuine laughter. Finally, while the statement in choice **d** may be true, the public laughter probably would not reflect an implication that the work was written for nonwriters.

9. b. Anderson discusses Stein's innovative use of words, emphasizing her use of small, everyday words that are often neglected by writers. The discussion of the frustration with language's limitations emphasizes Stein's ability to make the small words better, rather than her need to search for better words. He is not talking about the difficulties of writing in the context of Stein's relationship with her critics; that comes later. Nor is he self-reflexively discussing the passage essay itself, and the difficulty of writing it. While Anderson does mention the desire to create images in the mind of the reader, he does not entertain the possibility of a multimedia or image-based literature.

10. a. Anderson contrasts Stein's work with epic poetry and novels with grand ideas and describes Stein's work in terms of using little, underappreciated words. Here is a list of common everyday things. In paragraph 5, Anderson mentions "sonnets to my lady's eyes" in contrast to Stein's work, and while the line in choice **c** seems to discuss neglected citizens, Anderson uses the term "neglected citizens" as a metaphor to describe the types of words Stein uses—not her subject matter. Finally, "exultation" and "eternity" sound like grand ideas, which is in contrast to how Anderson describes Stein's work.

11. a. Anderson admires the way Stein uses the neglected everyday words in poetry (perhaps ones that would be found in a grocery list); many other critics at the time did not. Anderson does not mention rhyme or formal structure, or the Romantics, nor does his explanation seem to indicate that Stein does not use elegant words, but instead elevates common, ordinary words. But choice **c** focuses on the mixing of the elegant and the vulgar. If Anderson were responding to this critic, he might have agreed with him or her and then explained how this mix is innovative.

12. b. Anderson is very much focused on Stein's language. The entirety of paragraph 3 is a description of how he values the ability of words to create a sensory experience. Anderson does not write a great deal about Stein's life, except to say that she did not write novels or plays, and he does not incorporate her biography into an understanding of her poetry. He also does not really consider Stein's meaning but is rather focused on her language; he does not focus on the reader as meaning maker but instead focuses on the writer's perspective. Additionally, Anderson does not examine the structure of Stein's work, as he does not even provide an example of a single line.

13. d. Darwin focuses his discussion on processes like production and extinction and the interplay between diverse life forms in nature to posit how life changes over time through a process of natural selection. In the first sentence, Darwin states that many authors hold this view expressed in choice **a**, but the subject of these authors or their arguments is never revisited. He mentions gravity only once and does not go into detail about its effects on how various species developed over time, and while Darwin refers to beauty and perfection, his main goal is not to describe this aspect of life.

14. d. With these word choices, Darwin seeks to emphasize the elegance of the process of natural selection. Darwin mentions "the Creator" elsewhere in the text, but the overall passage argues a scientific phenomenon rather than divine creation, and in describing a process that involves a "war of nature," Darwin emphasizes through his word choice the elegance of this process rather than the savagery. Finally, while Darwin's descriptions seek to elevate species and the complex process they undergo, he does not go so far as to advocate that all species are in their "most perfect state."

15. b. Darwin makes a direct connection between "famine and death" (both things that sound bad) and the "most exalted object" (something that sounds good), implying irony. The fact that good things can stem from bad highlights his awe for the process of natural selection. In context, Darwin is using exaggerated language to highlight how awe inspiring the process of natural selection is, not to make a philosophical claim about the limitations of human cognition or the existence of higher powers beyond humankind. The "higher animals" he describes may likely be predators, but this is a logical inference made by the reader rather than something Darwin implies. When he discusses the "most exalted thing," he does not mean to exalt predators but rather describe more complex life forms. Finally, while someone could use Darwin's statement to make the argument laid out in choice **d** (or potentially to argue the opposite), it is not implied by the author. Darwin does not discuss the militarized proclivities of human society.

16. d. Darwin describes a similar process in the passage through small variances over a long period of time but does not have the terminology from contemporary genetic science. The process of natural selection as described by Darwin happens through a "war of nature," not through scientific experimentation, and Darwin at no point describes radical changes from species to their offspring, but rather a long slow process of transformation through natural selection. Finally, Darwin says that futurity will contain "larger and dominant groups, which will ultimately prevail and procreate new and dominant species," but he does not mean that the earth will only be populated by large animals in the future.

17. b. This answer describes a process similar to natural selection as described in the passage, except it is applied to ideas rather than species. The passage posits that species are not independently created but evolve over time. If ideas function as species do, then ideas do not originate independently in the brain but are influenced by external pressures as well as ideas of the past. Darwin discusses species of the far-distant future, but the logic of his argument does not apply to ideas. Finally, that all species are descended from one or a few original species is discussed by the author in the passage, but this is not a description of the process of natural selection; rather, it is the condition posited by the author that precedes natural selection.

18. c. Darwin states specifically, "of the species now living very few will transmit progeny of any kind to a far distant futurity." Endangered species today would not likely be among the "very few" that the author discusses, and while he discusses how all species undergo a "struggle for life," which would include endangered species, he does not take a stance on the morality of the process. Darwin emphasizes a beauty to the "production of higher animals" but does not emphasize the beauty of extinct species. Logically it would follow that he would not emphasize the beauty of species in danger of becoming extinct. And while he could agree that humans endanger other species, but it is not clear that he would claim that the human species is beyond the natural world.

19. d. Thoreau critiques convention and habit and emphasizes that one should be "obedient to the laws of his being" and advance "confidently in the direction of his dreams." He merely begins his discussion with Mirabeau and then moves on to discuss other subjects, mentions leaving the woods as part of a larger explanation of his personal philosophy, and uses the "cabin passage" as a metaphor and at no point discusses a real sea voyage. Finally, Thoreau implies that a just government is a rarity; however, the author's main focus is not on government laws.

20. b. Thoreau makes a connection between paths of the earth and the paths of the mind as being "impressible." In context, he likens highways to the "ruts of tradition and conformity," suggesting further that people tend to follow the same paths and may conform to the same ideas. The first part of the answer may sound correct, but the statement has nothing to do with evolution, while choice **c** treats the earth metaphor too literally and conflates pathways in the brain with "the paths, which the mind travels." Thoreau does not consider neural pathways or refer to different societies. Finally, Thoreau's main intention is not to insult those who follow tradition.

21. c. Thoreau uses this quote to demonstrate Mirabeau's attitude toward laws and following authority but argues that one should not simply oppose laws and authority but be governed by the "laws of his being." Thoreau does not discuss the use of militaries or Mirabeau's use of metaphor. And while choice **d** is Mirabeau's argument and a correct explication of his quote, Thoreau does not employ the quote simply to agree with what Mirabeau has said.

22. a. A civil rights activist is likely governed by "a more sacred law" if she opposes an unjust law like segregation. The hungry man finds himself in opposition to the law not because he believes it is unjust or believes in a greater, more sacred law, but out of desperation and hunger, while the driver has a reckless disregard for the law rather than a belief that it is unjust and the banker highlights ways to work around the law but has nothing to with a greater sense of self or purpose.

23. a. This choice most closely resembles the attitudes expressed in paragraph 2, where the author expresses his desire to "go before the mast and on the deck of the world, for there I could best see the moonlight amid the mountains." In paragraph 1, Thoreau mentions that Mirabeau disobeys authority simply to test his resolve and demonstrates his disagreement with this attitude, and when Thoreau discusses a sea voyage as a metaphor ("the deck of the world"), he says, "I do not wish to go below now." To stay belowdecks and keep to himself does not align with the attitude that he has "several more lives to live." Thoreau discusses conformity in paragraph 2 and has the attitude that a man should forge his own path, be obedient to the laws of his own being, and follow confidently in the direction of his dreams. Nonconformity is not simply for the sake of being unconventional but to make space for a greater sense of the self.

24. c. Thoreau emphasizes that an individual must be obedient to the laws of his being over any laws created by society. While he might agree that individuals are shaped by their experiences, he does not discuss the origin of the individual, so it is unclear whether he would agree that the individual begins as a blank slate, and he does not discuss a scientific notion of the self. Additionally, Thoreau places great stock in individuality and does not attempt to dismantle the self into thought processes.

25. b. Ruskin provides several examples of "magnificence" in architecture (the Parthenon, the Pyramid of Cheops, and St. Peter's) that would fit in well with the "colossal" Alps, while criticizing the small cottage that is out of sync with the scene. Ruskin criticizes the neatness of a specific piece of architecture (a cottage) when it does not suit the grandeur of its surrounding environment. This means not that neatness in itself is a bad quality but that it requires a more appropriate setting. And while he does discuss the offensiveness of the small cottage as it disrupts the natural scene, he offers other examples of architecture that would enhance the scene, so it is not simply that any building on the hillside would be offensive. Finally, the purpose of Ruskin's description of the natural scene is not to say that it is better than any piece of architecture—in fact he also admires several other architectural examples—but rather to criticize the small piece of architecture that exists in this natural scene in order to examine the relationship between structure and setting.

26. c. The metaphor emphasizes the smallness of the cottage, which, like a fallen toy, is not where it should be. Ruskin does not mention that the cottage is in need of repair, and elsewhere he even mentions the cottage's "neatness" and "ornamentation," although these features contribute to its unsightliness, and while choice **b** might seem like a logical choice because the cottage is being equated with a child's toy, perhaps equating the creator of the cottage to a child, the focus of the metaphor is the cottage rather than its creator. The entire passage discusses the aesthetics of the cottage in its setting without really mentioning the architect who put it there. Finally, Ruskin criticizes the cottage harshly throughout the passage. His level of attention could possibly be described as "fascinated," but the author by no means finds the cottage "wondrous," nor does he imply that all viewers would see it the same way.

27. a. Ruskin mentions these famous structures as examples of architecture that could match the beauty and magnitude of the setting of the Alps, saying that the visual effect of each would be enhanced by their juxtaposition. While Ruskin imagines these buildings in the setting of the Alps, their actual location is not discussed. And the mention of older, even ancient, structures is not to emphasize age, but to introduce famous references that the reader might know. The cottage is not discussed as an emblem of all modern architecture but used to discuss the way architecture and environment interact. Finally, Ruskin does not mention the building materials of these famous structures; he rather focuses on their proportions.

28. b. A skyscraper would look rather bizarre in a country lane; the setting would not enhance the beauty of the building nor vice versa, which is precisely what Ruskin rails against in the passage. The passage is all about the interplay between a building and its surrounding. Times Square is full of neon signs and advertisements, and a McDonald's would fit in appropriately with the city scene. The author mentions the Pyramid of Cheops in the passage as one example of a building of magnitude that could match the grandeur of the Alps; the scale of the Pyramid is enhanced by the vastness of the desert. Finally, Ruskin discusses examples of larger structures in the Alps that would look better than a tiny cottage, and a castle, which is considerably larger than a cottage, would probably not offend his sensibilities.

29. d. This is the larger point of the passage—that the small cottage is offensive to the eye because it is incongruous with the landscape around it. If Ruskin were to give advice, it would be that architects should strive to create work that enhances the landscape around it and vice versa. Choice **a** may be good advice, especially given Ruskin's harsh critique, but it does not speak to his intention or the real purpose of the passage, and while Ruskin's metaphor for the cottage is as "a child's toy let fall on the hillside," uses this metaphor primarily to portray the visual proportion of the cottage in the Alps rather than to suggest some architect treated his project recklessly. Finally, choice **c** is a very literal reading of the passage, instead of grasping a broader interpretation that can be applied to another situation. While Ruskin primarily discusses a cottage in the Alps in the passage, he discusses specifics of color, material, and size of the cottage as incongruous to the landscape. A cottage made to fit in with the landscape on a smaller hill could work better.

30. b. The quote sounds very similar to Ruskin's main point in the passage—that a piece of architecture should fit in with its setting and enhance it. The excerpt from Ruskin's work critiques the cottage as a piece of architecture but is too dismissive to consider the cottage an "artistic creation" and certainly does not consider the philosophy behind its creation the way Wright does. In the discussion of materials, Ruskin critiques the "neatness" and "weakness" of the deal boards (made of pine or fir) of the cottage, but it's unclear whether he finds the materials unappealing by themselves or only in contrast to the beauty of the natural materials around the cottage. He would certainly say the wood was not well used by the architect of the cottage, but choice **c** is too tenuous compared to choice **b**. Ruskin does not believe that building the cottage has glorified the wood at all but rather made it look "dead, raw, and lifeless."

31. d. All of these statements are examples from the third paragraph, where Tridon lists various aspects of Freud's theories of dream psychology. In this passage, Tridon discusses Freud's theory of wish fulfillment (I), but he also discusses Freud's connection between dreams and insanity (II), as well as the idea that dream visions are symbolic (III), and the the third choice is a statement that aligns with Freud's theories, but it is not the *only* one, and it is not *only* (I) and (II) that are correct.

32. c. Tridon says specifically that these psychologists' methods were not supported by evidence. Tridon does not discuss the emotions of these psychologists in his criticism, and the issues with these methods as discussed by Tridon have nothing to do with how the theories are communicated but relate to the nature of the theories themselves. Finally, while answer **d** sounds like something Tridon could say, elsewhere he uses the words "empty" and "artificial" to criticize this method of psychological theorizing. But in context, Tridon describes these methods as inventions, focusing particularly on the fact that they are not supported by evidence.

33. b. Minerva represents the birth of a hypothesis, and the "stretched hide" indicates that reality had to be killed to wrap it around the theoretical framework. Before Freud developed "the truth is what works," according to Tridon, many psychologists had theories that negated reality instead of reflecting it. Tridon is using a string of metaphors at this point in the text, which makes his meaning complex and confusing. Choice **a** attempts to take two separate metaphors and mash them into one. Minerva was not the goddess of war but of wisdom, and according to legend, she was born from her father's forehead. In the next

sentence, Tridon refers to "autistic ways" as a rigid frame that psychologists stretch their theories on. The metaphors are not particularly connected, and this answer choice does not help pinpoint the author's meaning. Tridon does not focus on psychologists' arrogance but rather the distortion of their ideas. The reference to the birth of Minerva refers to the psychologists' hypotheses rather than the psychologists themselves. And Tridon does not appear to believe that ideas that come from the brain become weakened under further consideration.

34. d. In trying to discuss Freud's use of empirical evidence, Tridon uses this colloquial phrase, which does not sound like a precise fact, so it does not sound like appropriate evidence for his argument. In the first paragraph, Tridon tries to explain Freud's use of empirical evidence for his theories by pointing out the time and consideration he employed to develop them, not with an emotional appeal. The use of quotations may be suspect because Tridon does not attribute the quote correctly or clarify whether he is in fact quoting Freud. But in describing Freud's methods, Freud's own statements would actually be useful. This piece of criticism used in choice **c** is vague rather than incisive. Tridon's phrasing is odd, but he is saying that Freud looked at the facts, rather than suggesting "ideas just came to him."

35. a. In the first paragraph, Tridon mentions that Freud did not have preconceived notions of his dream theory but instead observed evidence of patterns in his patients. This could be a response to accusations that Freud went looking for a specific pattern that matched his own experience. In the second and third paragraphs, Tridon discusses Freud's innovations, but the first paragraph seems to offer a defense of Freud as an observer, a statistician, and a collector of information who did not simply "invent" but created theory based on evidence. Tridon does not discuss how Freud dealt with criticism, so it does not seem that the passage would be a response to this accusation. The accusation leveled in choice **d** is tantamount to saying Freud was on drugs so his theories should be discarded. It does not go so far as to accuse Freud of "inventing" his theory based on hallucinations. If Tridon's explanation of Freud's "scientific method" in the first paragraph were in response to this accusation, he would probably have paid closer attention to Freud's own mental clarity.

36. c. Tridon discusses the relationship between sleeping states and waking states and the universality of dream symbols. If three people have the same dream, it is likely because the symbolism of the dream is universal and the dream indicates something going on in their daily lives. Tridon mentions Freud's idea that symbolic actions of the "mentally insane" mirror symbolic dream actions—which would suggest that an insane person might show up nude in inappropriate places in his or her waking life, rather than that the three dreamers suffer a mental illness. Choice **b** refers to Freud's theory of "wish fulfillment," but the passage also emphasizes that bizarre dream occurrences are actually symbolic, so being naked in a dream may actually have a symbolic meaning rather than express the literal desire to be an exhibitionist. Finally, Tridon discusses Freud's ideas that there is a universal symbolic dream language but at no point suggests that dreamers are psychically linked.

37. d. In the passage, Jacobs discusses examples of the Greeks' understanding of world geography, as well as their influences and the sources of their knowledge. Joseph Jacobs begins his discussion with the poems of Homer but moves on from there to discuss Greek colonization and maps. Jacobs discusses the influences the Babylonians had on the Greeks but still attributes the invention of map drawing to a Greek philosopher, Anaximander. Jacobs in no way "denounces" Greek colonization but rather discusses the facts of it without offering judgment on its rightness or wrongness.

38. c. Within the context of the sentence, the word "navel" means "center." Jacobs is primarily discussing location at this point. The word "navel" may be confused with "naval," which has to do with warships. Jacobs does not discuss how Greek colonies were dependent on Delphi, as the term "lifeline" suggests, but rather their concept of the entire world beyond Greece, and he does not discuss the origin of Greek civilization but rather their early concepts of geography.

39. d. The author says that Homer describes the location of pygmies—people who had been considered fictional until anthropologists later confirmed this knowledge. This strengthens the use of a poem as a means of discovering historical geographical knowledge regarding the areas Homer actually knew, i.e., "Northern Greece and of the western coasts of Asia Minor, some acquaintance with Egypt, Cyprus, and Sicily." Jacobs does not bring up the work of anthropologists in order to reach the conclusion that aspects of fables are real but rather to show that aspects of the work of Homer were factual, even when they had been disregarded as fabulous for a long time. And he does not object to applying the term "discovery" to a people, as the anthropologists were described as rediscovering the pygmies. Finally, from the context it is not clear that people regarded Homer as the creator of this fable. Furthermore, the mention of the anthropologists focuses on the fact that something considered fabulous actually turned out to be true.

40. a. If the oldest map of the world contained a cuneiform inscription, then it was not drawn by the Greek "inventor of map-drawing." Thus, mapmaking can possibly not be claimed as his "invention." (However, Jacobs possibly intended to go into the subtleties between cuneiform inscription, which involves using stick-like tools in clay, and "drawing," which more traditionally refers to some kind of pigment on paper.) Choice **b** would appear to strengthen Jacobs's final sentence inasmuch as providing a reason for a culture's invention of map-drawing, while choice **c** is irrelevant to the final sentence of the passage, and though Homer's concept of the world predates the first maps, it is an example of geographical knowledge that can be recorded without a map, so it does not really contradict Jacobs's statement.

41. c. Jacobs emphasizes that the Greeks were best known for their curiosity, and it is this quality that led them to obtain and record geographical information. Jacobs discusses the Greek colonies without reference to war or any details of the colonization except for the location of the colonies and does not mention the richness of the Greeks or sponsored explorations. And while he discusses the Greeks' conception of the location of the ocean, he does not discuss their access to ocean routes as affecting their ability to explore.

42. c. Russell initially calls into question the certainty of observations and assumed facts, discussing the difficulty of determining anything to be "true." The color of the table is an example used to elucidate Russell's ideas about appearance and reality. Determining the true color is not really Russell's purpose. In the final paragraph Russell discusses these differences, but in the initial paragraphs he does not. The painter is used as an example of a way one might see the world, and the overall discussion focuses on perception versus reality. And while Russell discusses the practical, he does not mention the fantastical.

43. c. In paragraph 2, Russell discusses how light changes the distribution of color on the table as a person moves. Choice **a** is similar to what Russell discusses in the first paragraph—doubting perception and what can be an agreed-upon fact—but the discussion of the table color is in paragraph 2, while Russell does not discuss the psychology of the viewers or how medical conditions affect perception.

44. b. The author takes pains to discuss different points of perception but does not doubt the person who perceives that these things really exist. While the author's language often refers to *men*, the discussion is not actually gendered. This might be an appropriate criticism of his word choice but not really of his argument. Meanwhile, choice **c** is dismissive of the author but does not actually tackle the argument he tries to make, and considering the table as a collection of atoms is another perspective on the table, which the author could use to bolster his doubt.

45. b. In the search for "certainty," Russell lists several observable facts in front of him but most likely references the specific distance to the sun to establish that even agreed-upon scientific data is called into question. The distance to the sun is not really relevant to the discussion of a person's perception of light reflecting off a table, and Russell does not connect the two things, and while Russell wants to establish things that any "normal" observer would agree with, the fact is not used to establish his own authority but rather to pick a fact that anyone might agree on. Finally, Russell does not define "normal" perception but takes that as a given. The distance to the sun alludes to another type of perception (i.e., that of the telescope), but he does not connect that with the painter's perception.

46. c. Russell's main point about the color of the table is that it changes with the viewer's perspective. This would be that case with the table's shape as well—the angles of the four corners would look different at different points in the room. Russell brings up the example of the painter in the last paragraph as someone who is really looking at the table, attempting to copy exactly what he sees, disregarding "common sense" that says the table is brown (or in the case of this question, a rectangular shape), but he does not conclude that the artist is able to determine the "true" nature of the table. Rather, he concludes that the artist captures only what "seems" to be. The practical human would likely want to know what shape the table really is, just as he wanted to know about its color, and Russell doubts the sense of touch as much as the sense of sight. The first paragraph demonstrates that doubt surrounds accepted facts of science and all appearances around him, including that he feels the table pressing against his arm.

47. a. Option I sounds logical, but it would contradict Russell's argument most directly. He brings up differing points of view of a single object as problematic, rather than as proof it exists. Option III concludes that we can know something is true, which Russell would certainly not agree with, since he continually questions whether we can truly know something. Choice **b** fits with what Russell is saying, so it is not a contradiction, whereas choice **c** contradicts Russell's statements, but is not the only option that contradicts him. Given Russell's statements about certainty, Option IV, which questions the very concept of certainty, does not contradict his arguments but rather opens up his discussion. Option II does not contradict the author's argument, either.

48. b. From the context of the sentence, a combustive nature is a sign of language that has not been "arrested by any literary interference." Once the language becomes written, it is in a fixed form. If it is only spoken, then it may constantly change and breed new dialects. From the context of the sentence, Müller's meaning is the opposite of choice **a**, there is no mention of the effectiveness of communication of different types of languages, and while choice **d** might be a synonym for combustion in another context, when "explosive" is applied to the term "language," it usually means "strong" language or "bad" language, which Müller does not mean.

49. b. There are several examples in the passage that pit dialects against literary language. Müller's use of the word "tyranny" suggests strongly that literary language has wrongfully taken prominence over the language of dialects. In the context of the passage, choice **a** does not really suggest bias; it is neither negative nor positive. Choice **c** refers to literary languages, but not in a negative way, and choice **d** refers to dialects, not literary language.

50. c. This is the correct answer. Müller cites Grimm in order to critique him and demonstrate why he believes quite the opposite—that dialects are the "feeders rather than the channels" of literary languages. The theories in choice **a** sound similar, but his theory isn't necessarily discredited, even if was inspired by the theory of evolution. The theory is possibly vulnerable to the criticism in choice **b**, but it is a debatable claim. Finally, Grimm's theory depends on the idea that a greater number of dialects are presently spoken, as it posits, "the more we look backward in the history of language the smaller."

51. b. Müller consistently advocates for the belief that dialects feed and shape languages that have risen to prominence. Elsewhere, Müller argues that literature arrests a language's development and does not ever mention transcribing dialects as a practice, does not use the term "logic" or appear to be tracing the rise of certain words' popularity—he rather discusses language and dialect in a broader sense—and wishes to undercut the idea that dialects are merely corruptions of a literary language, so it is unlikely that this is the term he sets out to define.

52. c. Müller specifically says in the first paragraph that in order to gain insight into the growth of languages, we must study the dialects of tribes who have no written language. Müller does not advocate that linguists should study dead languages but insists that a historian of language should study the literary languages he terms "dynasties" in addition to dialects. He also uses the term "corruption" to describe a specific type of dialect, not to object to the term but rather to support the idea that all dialects are corruptions. The study of literature is irrelevant to the passage.

53. b. Müller describes dialects as feeders and streams that run parallel to literary language. Müller does emphasize the growth of language, but choice **a** sounds similar to how Grimm conceives of dialects—that the multiplicity of dialects stem from a unified language—and Müller does not agree. Müller also emphasizes the changing nature of dialects, which runs counter to the idea of them being "firm" and "fixed," and does not emphasize the idea that dialects are indistinguishable from a larger language or are static, like sand on a beach.

4 ▶ MCAT® EXAM PRACTICE TEST 2

CHAPTER SUMMARY

This is the second of two practice MCAT® exams.

The exam is organized in four sections:

- Biological and Biochemical Foundations of Living Systems
- Chemical and Physical Foundations of Biological Systems
- Psychological, Social, and Biological Foundations of Behavior
- Critical Analysis and Reasoning Skills

(Note: you will have access to the Periodic Table of Elements during the exam.)

This practice test is modeled on the content, format, and length of the official MCAT® exam. At the beginning of each section you'll find the number of questions and the time allotted. We recommend that you take the test under timed conditions so you can get an accurate assessment of how you might do on test day and determine the pace you'll need to work at.

Use your results on each section of the exam to determine your strengths and weaknesses and guide your study. Good luck!

Part 1: Biological and Biochemical Foundations of Living Systems

1.	ⓐ ⓑ ⓒ ⓓ	21.	ⓐ ⓑ ⓒ ⓓ	41.	ⓐ ⓑ ⓒ ⓓ
2.	ⓐ ⓑ ⓒ ⓓ	22.	ⓐ ⓑ ⓒ ⓓ	42.	ⓐ ⓑ ⓒ ⓓ
3.	ⓐ ⓑ ⓒ ⓓ	23.	ⓐ ⓑ ⓒ ⓓ	43.	ⓐ ⓑ ⓒ ⓓ
4.	ⓐ ⓑ ⓒ ⓓ	24.	ⓐ ⓑ ⓒ ⓓ	44.	ⓐ ⓑ ⓒ ⓓ
5.	ⓐ ⓑ ⓒ ⓓ	25.	ⓐ ⓑ ⓒ ⓓ	45.	ⓐ ⓑ ⓒ ⓓ
6.	ⓐ ⓑ ⓒ ⓓ	26.	ⓐ ⓑ ⓒ ⓓ	46.	ⓐ ⓑ ⓒ ⓓ
7.	ⓐ ⓑ ⓒ ⓓ	27.	ⓐ ⓑ ⓒ ⓓ	47.	ⓐ ⓑ ⓒ ⓓ
8.	ⓐ ⓑ ⓒ ⓓ	28.	ⓐ ⓑ ⓒ ⓓ	48.	ⓐ ⓑ ⓒ ⓓ
9.	ⓐ ⓑ ⓒ ⓓ	29.	ⓐ ⓑ ⓒ ⓓ	49.	ⓐ ⓑ ⓒ ⓓ
10.	ⓐ ⓑ ⓒ ⓓ	30.	ⓐ ⓑ ⓒ ⓓ	50.	ⓐ ⓑ ⓒ ⓓ
11.	ⓐ ⓑ ⓒ ⓓ	31.	ⓐ ⓑ ⓒ ⓓ	51.	ⓐ ⓑ ⓒ ⓓ
12.	ⓐ ⓑ ⓒ ⓓ	32.	ⓐ ⓑ ⓒ ⓓ	52.	ⓐ ⓑ ⓒ ⓓ
13.	ⓐ ⓑ ⓒ ⓓ	33.	ⓐ ⓑ ⓒ ⓓ	53.	ⓐ ⓑ ⓒ ⓓ
14.	ⓐ ⓑ ⓒ ⓓ	34.	ⓐ ⓑ ⓒ ⓓ	54.	ⓐ ⓑ ⓒ ⓓ
15.	ⓐ ⓑ ⓒ ⓓ	35.	ⓐ ⓑ ⓒ ⓓ	55.	ⓐ ⓑ ⓒ ⓓ
16.	ⓐ ⓑ ⓒ ⓓ	36.	ⓐ ⓑ ⓒ ⓓ	56.	ⓐ ⓑ ⓒ ⓓ
17.	ⓐ ⓑ ⓒ ⓓ	37.	ⓐ ⓑ ⓒ ⓓ	57.	ⓐ ⓑ ⓒ ⓓ
18.	ⓐ ⓑ ⓒ ⓓ	38.	ⓐ ⓑ ⓒ ⓓ	58.	ⓐ ⓑ ⓒ ⓓ
19.	ⓐ ⓑ ⓒ ⓓ	39.	ⓐ ⓑ ⓒ ⓓ	59.	ⓐ ⓑ ⓒ ⓓ
20.	ⓐ ⓑ ⓒ ⓓ	40.	ⓐ ⓑ ⓒ ⓓ		

Part 2: Chemical and Physical Foundations of Biological Systems

1.	ⓐ ⓑ ⓒ ⓓ	21.	ⓐ ⓑ ⓒ ⓓ	41.	ⓐ ⓑ ⓒ ⓓ
2.	ⓐ ⓑ ⓒ ⓓ	22.	ⓐ ⓑ ⓒ ⓓ	42.	ⓐ ⓑ ⓒ ⓓ
3.	ⓐ ⓑ ⓒ ⓓ	23.	ⓐ ⓑ ⓒ ⓓ	43.	ⓐ ⓑ ⓒ ⓓ
4.	ⓐ ⓑ ⓒ ⓓ	24.	ⓐ ⓑ ⓒ ⓓ	44.	ⓐ ⓑ ⓒ ⓓ
5.	ⓐ ⓑ ⓒ ⓓ	25.	ⓐ ⓑ ⓒ ⓓ	45.	ⓐ ⓑ ⓒ ⓓ
6.	ⓐ ⓑ ⓒ ⓓ	26.	ⓐ ⓑ ⓒ ⓓ	46.	ⓐ ⓑ ⓒ ⓓ
7.	ⓐ ⓑ ⓒ ⓓ	27.	ⓐ ⓑ ⓒ ⓓ	47.	ⓐ ⓑ ⓒ ⓓ
8.	ⓐ ⓑ ⓒ ⓓ	28.	ⓐ ⓑ ⓒ ⓓ	48.	ⓐ ⓑ ⓒ ⓓ
9.	ⓐ ⓑ ⓒ ⓓ	29.	ⓐ ⓑ ⓒ ⓓ	49.	ⓐ ⓑ ⓒ ⓓ
10.	ⓐ ⓑ ⓒ ⓓ	30.	ⓐ ⓑ ⓒ ⓓ	50.	ⓐ ⓑ ⓒ ⓓ
11.	ⓐ ⓑ ⓒ ⓓ	31.	ⓐ ⓑ ⓒ ⓓ	51.	ⓐ ⓑ ⓒ ⓓ
12.	ⓐ ⓑ ⓒ ⓓ	32.	ⓐ ⓑ ⓒ ⓓ	52.	ⓐ ⓑ ⓒ ⓓ
13.	ⓐ ⓑ ⓒ ⓓ	33.	ⓐ ⓑ ⓒ ⓓ	53.	ⓐ ⓑ ⓒ ⓓ
14.	ⓐ ⓑ ⓒ ⓓ	34.	ⓐ ⓑ ⓒ ⓓ	54.	ⓐ ⓑ ⓒ ⓓ
15.	ⓐ ⓑ ⓒ ⓓ	35.	ⓐ ⓑ ⓒ ⓓ	55.	ⓐ ⓑ ⓒ ⓓ
16.	ⓐ ⓑ ⓒ ⓓ	36.	ⓐ ⓑ ⓒ ⓓ	56.	ⓐ ⓑ ⓒ ⓓ
17.	ⓐ ⓑ ⓒ ⓓ	37.	ⓐ ⓑ ⓒ ⓓ	57.	ⓐ ⓑ ⓒ ⓓ
18.	ⓐ ⓑ ⓒ ⓓ	38.	ⓐ ⓑ ⓒ ⓓ	58.	ⓐ ⓑ ⓒ ⓓ
19.	ⓐ ⓑ ⓒ ⓓ	39.	ⓐ ⓑ ⓒ ⓓ	59.	ⓐ ⓑ ⓒ ⓓ
20.	ⓐ ⓑ ⓒ ⓓ	40.	ⓐ ⓑ ⓒ ⓓ		

Part 3: Psychological, Social, and Biological Foundations of Behavior

1.	(a) (b) (c) (d)	21.	(a) (b) (c) (d)	41.	(a) (b) (c) (d)
2.	(a) (b) (c) (d)	22.	(a) (b) (c) (d)	42.	(a) (b) (c) (d)
3.	(a) (b) (c) (d)	23.	(a) (b) (c) (d)	43.	(a) (b) (c) (d)
4.	(a) (b) (c) (d)	24.	(a) (b) (c) (d)	44.	(a) (b) (c) (d)
5.	(a) (b) (c) (d)	25.	(a) (b) (c) (d)	45.	(a) (b) (c) (d)
6.	(a) (b) (c) (d)	26.	(a) (b) (c) (d)	46.	(a) (b) (c) (d)
7.	(a) (b) (c) (d)	27.	(a) (b) (c) (d)	47.	(a) (b) (c) (d)
8.	(a) (b) (c) (d)	28.	(a) (b) (c) (d)	48.	(a) (b) (c) (d)
9.	(a) (b) (c) (d)	29.	(a) (b) (c) (d)	49.	(a) (b) (c) (d)
10.	(a) (b) (c) (d)	30.	(a) (b) (c) (d)	50.	(a) (b) (c) (d)
11.	(a) (b) (c) (d)	31.	(a) (b) (c) (d)	51.	(a) (b) (c) (d)
12.	(a) (b) (c) (d)	32.	(a) (b) (c) (d)	52.	(a) (b) (c) (d)
13.	(a) (b) (c) (d)	33.	(a) (b) (c) (d)	53.	(a) (b) (c) (d)
14.	(a) (b) (c) (d)	34.	(a) (b) (c) (d)	54.	(a) (b) (c) (d)
15.	(a) (b) (c) (d)	35.	(a) (b) (c) (d)	55.	(a) (b) (c) (d)
16.	(a) (b) (c) (d)	36.	(a) (b) (c) (d)	56.	(a) (b) (c) (d)
17.	(a) (b) (c) (d)	37.	(a) (b) (c) (d)	57.	(a) (b) (c) (d)
18.	(a) (b) (c) (d)	38.	(a) (b) (c) (d)	58.	(a) (b) (c) (d)
19.	(a) (b) (c) (d)	39.	(a) (b) (c) (d)	59.	(a) (b) (c) (d)
20.	(a) (b) (c) (d)	40.	(a) (b) (c) (d)		

Part 4: Critical Analysis and Reasoning Skills

1.	(a) (b) (c) (d)	19.	(a) (b) (c) (d)	37.	(a) (b) (c) (d)
2.	(a) (b) (c) (d)	20.	(a) (b) (c) (d)	38.	(a) (b) (c) (d)
3.	(a) (b) (c) (d)	21.	(a) (b) (c) (d)	39.	(a) (b) (c) (d)
4.	(a) (b) (c) (d)	22.	(a) (b) (c) (d)	40.	(a) (b) (c) (d)
5.	(a) (b) (c) (d)	23.	(a) (b) (c) (d)	41.	(a) (b) (c) (d)
6.	(a) (b) (c) (d)	24.	(a) (b) (c) (d)	42.	(a) (b) (c) (d)
7.	(a) (b) (c) (d)	25.	(a) (b) (c) (d)	43.	(a) (b) (c) (d)
8.	(a) (b) (c) (d)	26.	(a) (b) (c) (d)	44.	(a) (b) (c) (d)
9.	(a) (b) (c) (d)	27.	(a) (b) (c) (d)	45.	(a) (b) (c) (d)
10.	(a) (b) (c) (d)	28.	(a) (b) (c) (d)	46.	(a) (b) (c) (d)
11.	(a) (b) (c) (d)	29.	(a) (b) (c) (d)	47.	(a) (b) (c) (d)
12.	(a) (b) (c) (d)	30.	(a) (b) (c) (d)	48.	(a) (b) (c) (d)
13.	(a) (b) (c) (d)	31.	(a) (b) (c) (d)	49.	(a) (b) (c) (d)
14.	(a) (b) (c) (d)	32.	(a) (b) (c) (d)	50.	(a) (b) (c) (d)
15.	(a) (b) (c) (d)	33.	(a) (b) (c) (d)	51.	(a) (b) (c) (d)
16.	(a) (b) (c) (d)	34.	(a) (b) (c) (d)	52.	(a) (b) (c) (d)
17.	(a) (b) (c) (d)	35.	(a) (b) (c) (d)	53.	(a) (b) (c) (d)
18.	(a) (b) (c) (d)	36.	(a) (b) (c) (d)		

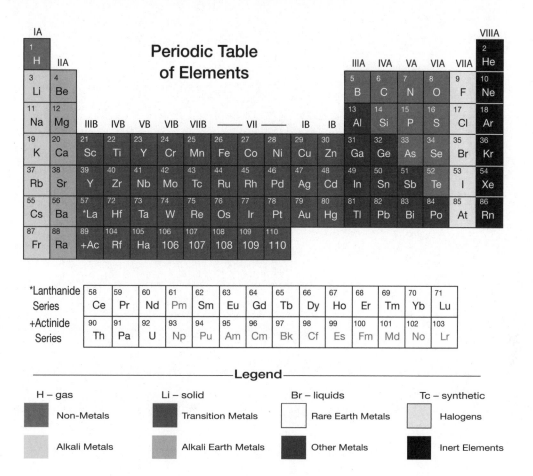

Periodic Table of Elements

Legend

H – gas	Li – solid	Br – liquids	Tc – synthetic
Non-Metals	Transition Metals	Rare Earth Metals	Halogens
Alkali Metals	Alkali Earth Metals	Other Metals	Inert Elements

Part 1: Biological and Biochemical Foundations of Living Systems

95 Minutes
59 Questions

Use the following passage to answer questions 1 through 4.

Very few proteins carry out their functions in the cell as unmodified folded polypeptides. Nearly all proteins undergo post-translational modifications (PTMs) in various cellular compartments, including the cytosol, Golgi apparatus, and endoplasmic reticulum. One common modification type is proteolytic cleavage, which involves irreversible processing of a polypeptide by proteases. Another major category of PTMs is covalent modification of specific amino acid residues. Among the many examples of these modifications are phosphorylation, acetylation, methylation, and glycosylation. There is evidence that every amino acid residue can be decorated with one or more of these modification groups. The specificity of this type of PTM is partially determined by the pattern of amino acids surrounding the target residue. Because PTMs affect myriad properties of proteins, including stability, localization, and interaction with other proteins, there has been intense effort in biological research to characterize the PTMs of individual proteins and protein populations in the cell. The influence of PTMs on protein function is illustrated by the example of p53, a canonical tumor suppressor protein. The levels of p53 in mammalian cells are tightly regulated by a modification called ubiquitination. Under normal conditions, the addition of multiple ubiquitin groups to p53 results in the sequestration of the protein into the 26S proteasome complex and its consequent clearance

from the cell. However, when the cell encounters stress, such as DNA damage or the activation of an oncogene, another pattern of PTM confers the stabilization of p53. Under these conditions, ubiquitination is suppressed, and p53 is instead acetylated and phosphorylated; both of these modifications stabilize the protein. P53 primarily functions as a transcriptional activator or repressor, and its target genes are involved in cell cycle arrest, apoptosis, and DNA repair. It accomplishes these functions in homotetrameric complexes, and phosphorylation of p53 has additionally been demonstrated to increase the complex's sequence-specific binding to DNA. PTMs are dynamic; phosphorylation, which often occurs in the cytosol, is controlled by kinase enzymes, whereas removal of phosphate groups is carried out by another set of enzymes called phosphatases. Similarly, while histone acetyltransferases add acetyl groups to p53, histone deacetylases remove them. P53 has also been shown to undergo additional PTMs: neddylation, which could repress its transactivator activity; sumoylation, which could act like ubiquitination; glycosylation; and ribosylation. The importance of p53 in cancer formation is illustrated by the fact that more than 20,000 mutations in the protein have been found in various cancer types. Many mutations lie in the p53 DNA binding domain and give rise to oncogenic properties. Additionally, mutations often result in increased phosphorylation and acetylation and, thus, stabilization of these oncogenic forms of p53.

1. Which of the following post-translational modifications is most likely to mark a protein for degradation?
   a. Monoubiquitination
   b. Polyubiquitination
   c. Acetylation
   d. Neddylation

2. Which of the following is a property of the cellular compartment where protein phosphorylation often occurs?
  a. It is aqueous.
  b. It is usually only found in eukaryotes.
  c. It has a pH of 6.5.
  d. It precipitates away from the other cellular compartments by high-speed centrifugation.

3. Which of the following is NOT a true similarity between covalent modifications and proteolytic cleavage?
  a. Both processes affect the cellular function of proteins.
  b. Both processes are controlled by enzymes.
  c. Both processes are reversible.
  d. Both processes affect protein localization.

4. Which method would likely NOT allow for the detection of different modification states of a protein?
  a. Deletion of an amino acid that bears the modification
  b. Mass spectrometry
  c. 2D gel electrophoresis
  d. Restriction enzyme digest

5. Which of the following amino acids is typically modified with a phosphate group?
  a. Proline
  b. Serine
  c. Tryptophan
  d. Valine

Use the following passage to answer questions 6 through 10.

Glucokinase possesses several properties that make it an attractive target for type 2 diabetes therapy, and several activators of the enzyme are currently being developed as potential drug candidates. Although there are numerous treatment options for type 2 diabetes, none of them allow for long-lasting control of blood glucose in most patients. Glucokinase, also known as hexokinase IV, is expressed in the liver and mediates the clearance of glucose from the blood through at least two different mechanisms. First, it catalyzes the phosphorylation of glucose to glucose 6-phosphate. Other forms of hexokinase (hexokinase I, II, III) catalyze the same reaction in other cells of the body, such as muscle cells. Second, glucokinase controls the levels of glucose by regulating the conversion of glucose to the storage form of glycogen. There is also evidence that glucokinase acts as a glucose sensor in pancreatic cells, where it is differentially expressed in response to glucose. These research observations led to speculation that glucokinase might be an important determinant of the diabetes phenotype. Indeed, family studies in the 1990s revealed that mutations associated with reduced glucokinase activity were associated with a form of diabetes known as maturity onset diabetes of the young (MODY). Furthermore, there is evidence that inactivating mutations act in a dose-dependent fashion: mutations in a single allele are linked to mild hyperglycemia, whereas homozygous mutations are linked to severe permanent diabetes in the neonatal stages. On the other hand, activating mutations have been found to cause hypoglycemia. The discovery of an allosteric site in glucokinase outside of its active site paved the way for the development of enzymatic activators starting in the early 2000s. In a recent study of patients with type 2 diabetes, one such activator was found to lower blood glucose. To date, numerous glucokinase activators have been developed, and their amino acid sequence may help lead to the identification of endogenous activators of the enzyme. In contrast, there is a physiologic negative allosteric effector of glucokinase, called fructose 6-phosphate, which is a product of the glycolytic pathway downstream of glucose 6-phosphate. Fructose 6-phosphate causes glucokinase to bind more tightly to a regulatory protein that sequesters the enzyme in the nucleus when blood glucose is low. However, when blood glucose is in the normal range, glucokinase dissociates from this regulatory protein, helping to keep the levels of glucose in the appropriate physiological range.

6. Within the glycolytic pathway, glucokinase catalyzes
   a. the first step.
   b. the second step.
   c. the sixth step.
   d. the tenth (and final) step.

7. How are hexokinase I and glucokinase (hexokinase IV) related to each other?
   a. They are homologs.
   b. They are orthologs.
   c. They are coenzymes.
   d. They are isozymes.

8. In addition to glycolysis, hepatic glucokinase also plays a key role in
   a. glycogenolysis.
   b. glycogenesis.
   c. gluconeogenesis.
   d. fermentation.

9. Which of the following is NOT true about allosteric effector molecules?
   a. They bind their substrate protein outside of its active site.
   b. They induce a conformational change in their substrate.
   c. They interact with their substrate through covalent binding.
   d. They can either activate or repress depending on the effector-substrate pair.

10. Based on the following graph, how do the Michaelis-Menten kinetics of hexokinase I and glucokinase differ from each other?

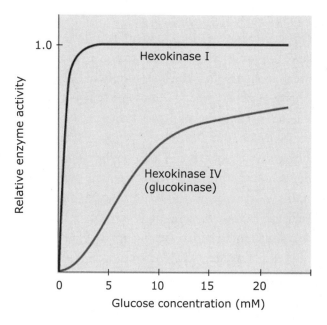

a. Hexokinase I has a higher K_m for glucose than glucokinase.
b. Glucokinase has a higher K_m for glucose than hexokinase I.
c. Hexokinase I has a higher V_{max} for glucose than glucokinase.
d. Glucokinase has a higher affinity for glucose than hexokinase I.

Use the following passage to answer questions 11 through 13.

An operon is a cluster of contiguous genes controlled by a single promoter and a regulatory element called the *operator*, which usually lies downstream from the promoter. The genes in an operon typically have related functions. The classic example of an operon, and the first to be characterized, is the lac operon in *E. coli*. The lac operon is composed of a promoter element (P); three operators (Os), termed O_1, O_2, and O_3; and three genes, *lacZ*, *lacY*, and *lacA*, which encode, respectively, β-galactosidase, β-galactoside permease, and β-galactoside transacetylase. Outside of the operon, the I gene encodes the lac repressor; in the absence of lactose, the lac repressor, as a tetrameric complex, binds the operators, blocking RNA polymerase transcription of *lacZ*, *lacY*, and *lacA*. As a result, these genes are expressed at low levels, giving rise to a baseline amount of enzymatic activity. However, when lactose is present outside the cell, the baseline level of β-galactoside permease pumps lactose into the cell, and β-galactosidase converts it to allolactose. Allolactose binds the repressor, resulting in its release from the operators. In this way, the lac operon is controlled by a positive feedback: lactose increases expression of *lacZ* and *lacY*, which in turn increases the uptake of lactose into cells. However, other energy sources also affect the induction of the lac operon. In the presence of a glucose, which is a more efficient energy source than lactose, the lac operon is repressed through a regulator protein called catabolite activator protein (CAP) and cyclic AMP (cAMP). The components of the lac operon were all originally identified through mutations, such as in the I gene (I^-), the promoter (P^-), and the operator elements ($O-$) that affected expression of *lacZ*, *lacY*, and *lacA*.

11. Which of the following statements about operons is NOT true?

   a. They are present in both prokaryotes and eukaryotes.

   b. The promoter and operon can overlap.

   c. Genes in an operon are coordinately transcribed.

   d. The proteins encoded by genes in an operon are always produced at equal molar levels.

12. Which type of operon is the lac operon?

   a. Positive inducible

   b. Negative inducible

   c. Repressible

   d. Constitutive

13. What is the predicted effect of the following genotype on expression of *lacZ*, *lacY*, and *lacA* (where + signifies wild-type)?

$$\frac{I^+ \; P^+ \; O^- \; lacZ^+ \; lacY^+ \; lacA^+}{I^+ \; P^+ \; O^+ \; lacZ^- \; lacY^- \; lacA^-}$$

   a. There would be constitutive expression of the genes.

   b. There would be repressed (baseline) expression of the genes.

   c. There would be no expression of the genes.

   d. There would be no effect on the expression of the genes.

Use the following information to answer questions 14 through 16.

A method termed *rapid amplification of cDNA ends* (RACE) was developed in the late 1980s to allow for the easy and fast generation of full-length complementary DNA (cDNA) copies of low-abundance messenger RNA molecules (mRNAs). In the first step, which relies on a unique property of mRNA, reverse transcriptase is employed to produce negative-strand cDNA from mRNA. This strand then serves as a template for the production of positive-strand cDNA. Finally, polymerase chain reaction (PCR) of the two strands results in the amplification of cDNA. The RACE method can be used in situations where only a partial sequence of mRNA is known and also to identify alternative gene transcripts. The technique can also be modified to create cDNA libraries from a pool of mRNA molecules.

The following figure illustrates the RACE method:

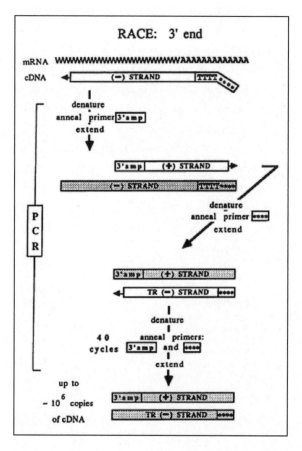

M. A. Frohman et al. Rapid production of full-length cDNAs from rare transcripts: amplification using a single gene-specific oligonucleotide primer. *Proc Natl Acad Sci*. 1988;85(23):8998–9002.

14. Based on the figure, the RACE method relies on which of the following mRNA modifications?
   a. 5' capping
   b. Splicing
   c. Polyadenylation
   d. Editing

15. How is RACE different from PCR?
   a. It requires a set of primers that are complementary to the nucleotide templates.
   b. It requires dNTPs to synthesize new DNA strands.
   c. It involves multiple cycles of denaturation, annealing, and elongation.
   d. It requires the reverse transcriptase enzyme.

16. Which of the following methods would NOT allow for the detection of alternatively spliced transcripts after conducting RACE?
   a. 2D gel electrophoresis
   b. Cloning and sequencing
   c. Northern blotting
   d. Southern blotting

Use the following information to answer questions 17 through 20.

Genes that are located on different chromosomes assort independently. However, genes on the same chromosome can still separate from each other through a process called recombination. During meiosis, when four homologous chromatids form a tetrad, two of the chromatids can cross over, which causes them to break from their chromatid and reattach to the other chromatid. When this crossover event happens between non-sister chromatids that contain different alleles of a gene, recombination takes place and gives rise to genetic diversity. Furthermore, the event can happen at more than one point between chromatids, resulting in multiple crossovers. Evidence of crossovers can be seen microscopically by the detection of chiasmata. These structures are thought to remain at the site of crossovers because the chromatids stay tangled together as the cell continues through meiosis. In addition to the detection of chiasmata, geneticists can identify crossover events by tracking the recombination of alleles on either side of the chromatid exchange. This tracking also allows the mapping of distance between genes. There is a direct correlation between the extent of recombination between two linked genes and their distance from each on a chromosome: genes that are far apart recombine frequently. The rates of recombination can also reveal the order of genes on a chromosome because single crossover events are much more likely to occur than multiple crossover events.

17. In a cross between a heterozygous *Drosophila* female (AB/ab) and a homozygous male (ab/ab), the frequency of progeny is as follows: 37 AB/ab, 46 ab/ab, 11 aB/ab, 7 Ab/ab. Based on these frequencies, what is the distance in centimorgan (cM) between genes a and b?
   a. 4 cM
   b. 7 cM
   c. 11 cM
   d. 18 cM

18. The table below shows the number of progeny from a cross between a *Drosophila* female that is heterozygous for three X-linked genes—a wing gene called crossveinless (cv), an eye gene called echinus (ec), and bristle gene called scute (sc)—with a male that has a mutant copy of each gene on his X chromosome. The genes are named for the phenotypes associated with their mutant forms. Because the wild-type (WT) genes are dominant, the female exhibits normal wings, eyes, and bristles; the male has the crossveinless, echinus, scute phenotypes. Based on the frequency of phenotypes among the progeny, what is the order of the genes on X chromosome?

PHENOTYPE	NUMBER OF PROGENY
wild-type	1,455
crossveinless, echinus, scute	1,158
crossveinless	148
echinus, scute	192
crossveinless, echinus	130
scute	163
crossveinless, scute	1
echinus	1

   a. cv-ec-sc
   b. cv-sc-ec
   c. ec-sc-cv
   d. sc-ec-cv

19. During which stage of meiosis does crossover between homologous chromosomes occur?
   a. Prophase of meiosis I
   b. Metaphase of meiosis I
   c. Prophase of meiosis II
   d. Metaphase of meiosis II

20. The two images below are of a chromosome pair, stained either with DAPI (to visualize the DNA) or HTP-3 (to visualize chromosomal axes), in wild-type *C. elegans* (top image) or in animals in which a protein that plays an important role in resolving crossovers, syp-1, was depleted (bottom image).

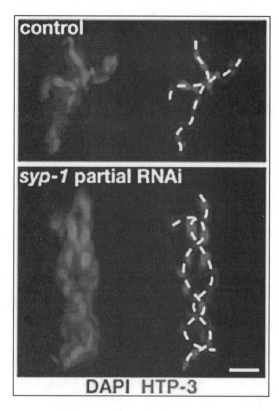

http://openi.nlm.nih.gov/detailedresult.php?img=3920622_nihms-516707-f0001&query=chiasma&it=xg&req=4&npos=28.

Based on the images, what is the difference in the number of chiasmata between the WT and syp-1–depleted animals?

a. The WT image has one more chiasmata than the syp-1–depleted image.

b. The syp-1–depleted image has four more chiasmata than the WT image.

c. The syp-1–depleted image has five more chiasmata than the WT image.

d. The WT and syp-1–depleted images have the same number of chiasmata.

Use the following information to answer questions 21 through 25.

HIV type 1 is one of several sexually transmitted infections, along with human papillomavirus and herpes simplex virus 2, that disproportionately affects women. Young women are an especially vulnerable population and represent more than 25% of new infections. In sub-Saharan Africa, which is the epicenter of the global HIV epidemic, women account for approximately 60% of people living with HIV. In addition to gender inequalities, there are biological factors that put women at a higher risk of being infected with HIV and change the course of disease, including anatomical and hormonal differences and X and Y chromosome–linked genes. Women actually have lower viral load and higher $CD4^+$ T-cell count than men in both acute and chronic infection; however, despite these factors, women experience faster disease progression and are more likely than men to develop AIDS. One of the major determinants of disease progression is immune activation. Plasmacytoid dendritic cells (pDCs) detect HIV-1 RNA via cell-surface molecules called Toll-like receptors (TLRs), of which there are about a dozen types in mammals. TLR-3, -7, and -8 recognize molecular patterns in RNA viruses, whereas TLR-4, -5, and -9 generally recognize ligands present in bacteria. In response, pDCs produce interferon-α (IFN-α), an antiviral cytokine molecule. Studies have reported that pDCs derived from women produce more IFN-α following exposure to HIV-1 than cells from men. Furthermore, one study found that a type of estrogen hormone, called 17-beta-estradiol, could boost the response of pDCs to HIV-1 exposure, which in turn could help mount a stronger immune response. The superior immune activation could, however, lead to a larger burden of non–AIDS-related disease, such as premature aging, in HIV-infected women, compared with men. Studies based on large health registries suggest that the increased risk of myocardial infarction associated with HIV-1 infection is greater for women than it is for men. More generally, sex-based differences in immune stimulation and the interferon-alpha response could put women at higher risk of various chronic and autoimmune diseases. Treatment with antiretroviral therapy (ART) appears to benefit women and men equally, although there are gender and racial differences in likelihood of starting ART. In addition, there are sex-based differences in the frequency of adverse events associated with ART, with women being at higher risk of developing nausea, skin rash, and other problems, while men are more likely to experience nausea and sleep difficulties.

21. Which of the following statements about interferons is NOT true?
    a. Interferon-α and -β are type I (antiviral) interferons.
    b. Plasmacytoid dendritic cells are a specialized cell type for producing interferon-α and -β.
    c. Interferon-κ is expressed in skin cells in response to viral infection.
    d. Interferon-γ is a type II interferon that does not have antiviral properties.

22. Scientists can experimentally determine whether TLR types 7 and 9 are important for stimulating IFN-α production by exposing cells to agonists of TLR7 or TLR9, called R848 and CpG, respectively. Based on the following graph, what can be concluded about the roles of TLR7 and TLR9?

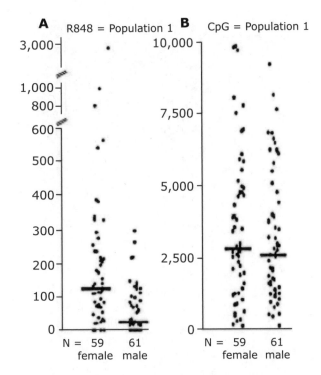

B. Berghöfer et al. TLR7 ligands induce higher IFN-alpha production in females. *J Immunol.* 2006;177(4):2088-2096. Copyright 2006. The American Association of Immunologists, Inc.

    a. The increased production of IFN-α in females compared with males is dependent on TLR7.
    b. The increased production of IFN-α in females compared with males is dependent on TLR9.
    c. The increased production of IFN-α in males compared with females is dependent on TLR7.
    d. The increased production of IFN-α in females compared with males is inhibited by TLR7.

23. The progesterone hormone has been shown to modulate the production of IFN-α in response to exposure to HIV-1 genomic RNA. Based on the following graph, which group of women would mount the strongest innate immune response to HIV-1 infection?

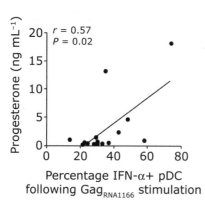

http://www.ncbi.nlm.nih.gov/pmc/articles/PMC2821111/.

 a. Postmenopausal women
 b. Women who have stopped taking combination birth control
 c. Women in the luteal phase of their menstrual cycle
 d. Women in the follicular phase of their menstrual cycle

24. Based on the table of hazard ratios (HRs) of time to initiation of ART, what conclusion can be made about the likelihood that the different groups will start therapy?

RACE AND SEX	HR	95% CI	P VALUE
White men	1.0	Reference	Reference
White women	1.38	(1.02–1.96)	0.056
Nonwhite men	0.78	(0.34–0.82)	0.003
Nonwhite women	0.45	(0.64–0.88)	0.004

 a. White men and nonwhite men have similar likelihoods of starting ART.
 b. White women are significantly more likely than white men to start ART.
 c. Nonwhite women are significantly less likely than white men to start ART.
 d. Nonwhite men and women have similar likelihoods of starting ART.

25. Which of the following diseases would NOT be predicted to disproportionately afflict women compared with men due to their stronger IFN-α response?
 a. Cardiovascular disease
 b. Hepatitis C virus infection
 c. Systemic lupus erythematosus
 d. Rheumatoid arthritis

Use the following passage to answer questions 26 through 32.

Mitochondria are thought to play a key regulatory role in the development of neurodegenerative disease and other age-related pathology. The organelle is the main source of ATP for the cell and is also involved in numerous processes, including phospholipid biosynthesis and calcium signaling. However, the process that forms ATP, termed *oxidative phosphorylation*, requires the transfer of electrons from food-derived molecules to oxygen and results in the production of reactive oxygen species (ROS). Indeed, most ROS are due to mitochondrial respiration. An estimated 1% to 2% of oxygen that is taken up by the body is turned into these radical species. Out of likely necessity, eukaryotic cells have evolved ample defense mechanisms to protect themselves from oxidative damage, including several mitochondrial antioxidant factors. Yet cellular insults can overcome the mechanisms for removing these species, resulting in a net gain in ROS. Oxidative stress can damage mitochondrial DNA (mtDNA), such as by causing double- and single-strand breaks, which are potentially mutagenic. Additional casualties of oxidative damage are mitochondrial proteins, some of which play important roles in the citric acid cycle upstream of oxidative phosphorylation and, thus, the generation of ATP. The depletion of ATP associated with ROS can lead to the induction of necrosis or to caspase-mediated apoptosis. Several lines of evidence suggest that mutations in mtDNA, which may result from oxidative stress, can cause age-related pathology. Mice that are genetically engineered to accumulate these mutations have phenotypes associated with early-onset aging: weight loss, alopecia, sarcopenia, and gonadal atrophy. Furthermore, analyses of the degenerated tissue in these animals revealed elevated levels of activated caspase enzymes that are markers for apoptosis. There is also mounting evidence that oxidative damage, as well as defenses against such damage, is associated with aging. Transcriptional analysis of postmortem brain samples from individuals ranging from ages 26 to 106 revealed, starting at around age 40, a decrease in expression of genes involved in mitochondrial function and an increase in stress-response, antioxidant, and DNA repair genes. Beyond normal aging, mitochondrial mutations and oxidative stress have been implicated in Alzheimer's disease, Parkinson's disease, and other neurodegenerative disorders. Experimental damage to the mitochondria is associated with Alzheimer's-like pathology in cells in vitro, such as increased amyloid-β peptide levels, and in animal models. A transgenic mouse that is deficient in the mitochondrial antioxidant enzyme manganese superoxide dismutase (MnSOD) developed amyloid-β plaques in the brain. Moreover, a number of disease-associated proteins, such as amyloid-β, amyloid precursor protein (APP), and parkin, which is associated with Parkinson's disease, have been found to interact with the mitochondria. However, these lines of evidence raise many new questions. For example, it is unclear why certain tissues are affected by mitochondrial mutations more than others, although it has been speculated that those with the highest energy demand are also the most susceptible to genetic aberrations. Furthermore, many questions remain about the potential of antioxidant treatment to affect the prognosis of age-related pathology. Thus far, clinical trials in which one or several antioxidants are given have reported little benefit. It remains possible that a more complex strategy for antioxidant therapy would be more beneficial.

26. Which of the following factors would NOT be expected to help protect mitochondria from oxidative damage?
   a. MnSOD
   b. Staurosporine
   c. Ubiquinone
   d. Vitamin E

27. The following illustration depicts the final stages of the oxidation of food molecules, including the citric acid cycle, or Krebs cycle, and oxidative phosphorylation.

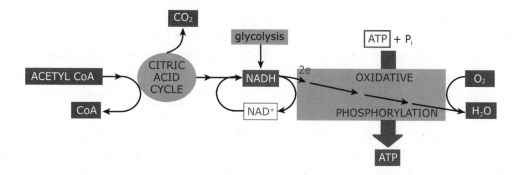

In which cellular compartment do these steps take place in eukaryotes?

a. Cytosol
b. Endoplasmic reticulum
c. Mitochondria
d. Nucleus

28. Which molecule in the illustration possesses the highest energy?
a. Acetyl-CoA
b. CO_2
c. NADH
d. NAD

29. Which of the following is NOT a similarity between apoptosis and necrosis?
a. They are both triggered by ROS production.
b. They both lead to cell death.
c. They are both mediated by caspase enzymes.
d. They are both associated with a rapid loss of cell membrane electrochemical potentials.

30. Based on the following reaction in oxidative phosphorylation depicting the conversion of O_2 to H_2O, which species is the first ROS intermediate?

$$O_2 \rightarrow O_2^- \rightarrow H_2O_2 \rightarrow OH \rightarrow H_2O$$

a. Oxygen
b. Superoxide anion
c. Hydrogen peroxide
d. Hydroxyl radical

31. Which experimental tool would help determine whether mutations in mtDNA cause age-related diseases?
a. Defective mutant in the proofreading activity of mtDNA polymerase
b. Defective mutant in the polymerase activity of mtDNA polymerase
c. RNA interference targeting the polymerase activity of mtDNA polymerase
d. RNA interference targeting mitochondrial transfer RNA (tRNA)

32. Which tissue type is predicted to be the least likely to develop disease as a result of mitochondrial mutations?
a. Brain
b. Gastrointestinal
c. Heart
d. Skeletal muscle

Use the following information to answer questions 33 through 38.

The epithelial cells of the oral, digestive, respiratory, and urinary tracts are the target cell type of many viruses, bacteria, and other pathogenic microorganisms. These cells are polarized, meaning their plasma membranes are divided into distinct apical (top) and basolateral (bottom) regions that feature distinct sets of cell surface proteins. This quality is an important early-defense cellular mechanism against infection. For example, several viruses depend on host factors for cell entry that are located in a plasma membrane domain to which circulating viruses do not have access. In addition to viruses, polarized cells restrict the passage of ions, solutes, and macromolecules across the epithelium. Cell polarity is created through the specific sorting, trafficking, and retention of proteins to their appropriate membrane domains. Junctions where neighboring cells interact with each other, via transmembrane proteins, create barriers that are also essential for polarity. In the complex tissue architecture, the apical domain faces the lumen, whereas the basolateral side is in contact with the extracellular matrix. Actin filaments, which are part of the cytoskeleton, are associated with the apical domain; they also help block viruses from entering the cell and are important for maintaining polarity. The filaments directly interact with the intracellular domain of transmembrane proteins involved in cell junctions. Given the fact that cell junction proteins are inaccessible from the extracellular space, it seems paradoxical that many viruses, including coxsackievirus, hepatitis C virus (HCV), and rotavirus, would specifically require these proteins. Yet a theme is emerging from years of research: viruses manage to make their way to junction proteins in a step-wise cell entry process. In the example of coxsackievirus, virions bind first to apically located cell surface protein, and this binding weakens the cellular transepithelial resistance (a measure of polarity) and helps bring the virion to another entry factor that is normally situated in hard-to-reach cell junctions. Following the association with junction proteins, the virion is endocytosed into the cell in a complex that includes these proteins. Similarly, in the early steps of HCV cell entry, virions bind to receptors that are normally accessible, and this association results in the translocation of virions to cell junctions, where they are endocytosed. Not surprisingly, the process of viral entry appears to disrupt polarity. Although the disruption is temporary and the epithelium likely recovers its polarized state, the loss is responsible for symptoms associated with infection. For example, rotavirus is the most common cause of severe gastroenteritis among young children globally. As the virions enter the gastrointestinal epithelium, they disrupt the integrity of cell junctions and the actin cytoskeleton, resulting in increased permeability across cells. These changes can be induced not just by virions but also by individual viral proteins and are sufficient to cause diarrhea, the hallmark characteristic of infection, in mice.

33. Which of the following is NOT a major function of actin filaments?
   a. Establish polarity
   b. Transport organelles across the cell
   c. Help stabilize microvilli
   d. Defend against viral infection

34. What is the name of the cell junction where the transmembrane proteins occludin and claudin are localized in the following illustration?

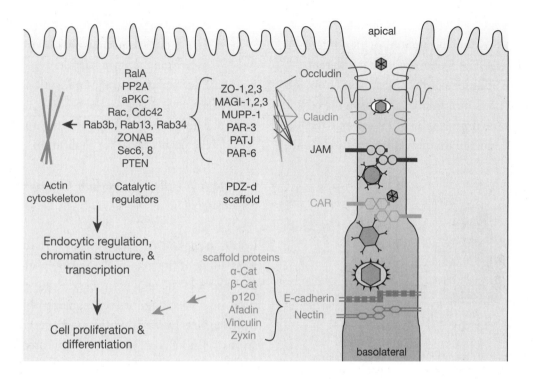

a. Adherens junction
b. Desmosomes
c. Gap junction
d. Tight junction

35. Which polarized cell domain would HCV and rotavirus virions be expected to use to enter their respective host cells?
a. HCV: apical; rotavirus: basolateral
b. HCV: apical; rotavirus: apical
c. HCV: basolateral; rotavirus: apical
d. HCV: basolateral; rotavirus: basolateral

36. Which of the following proteins would NOT be expected to disrupt cell polarity?
a. Cell junction protein with a defective extracellular domain
b. Cell junction protein with a defective actin binding site
c. Extracellular fragment of cell junction protein expressed in cells
d. Extracellular fragment of cell junction protein added to cell culture media

37. The following graph shows the results of an experiment using molecules that antagonize the function of cell surface proteins SRB1 and CD81, which HCV uses to enter cells. The y-axis represents the amount of viral infectivity in the cells. The six bars represent different times of additions of the antagonists (from left to right): before addition of virus to the cells, at the same time as virus addition, and 15, 30, 60, 120, and 240 minutes after virus addition.

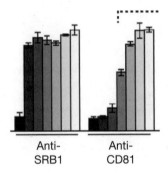

M. Sourisseau et al. Temporal analysis of hepatitis C virus cell entry with occludin directed blocking antibodies. *PLoS Pathog.* 2013;9(3):e1003244.

Based on the graph, what can be concluded about the roles of SRB1 and CD81 in HCV host cell entry?

a. HCV cell entry is step-wise, and the virus binds to CD81 first and then to SRB1.

b. HCV cell entry is step-wise, and the virus binds to SRB1 first and then to CD81.

c. HCV cell entry requires SRB1, but CD81 is only involved after virions have entered the cell.

d. HCV cell entry requires SRB1, but CD81 is not involved.

38. Which of the following statements about viral cell entry through endocytosis is NOT true?

a. Viruses can use several different endocytic pathways to enter the cell.

b. The endocytic pathway helps viruses overcome the actin barrier.

c. Encapsulation in the endocytic organelle makes it easier for the cell to detect the virus.

d. The low pH of the endocytic organelle helps the virus uncoat for replication.

Use the following information to answer questions 39 through 41.

Prions in the cell are synonymous with disease. Misfolding of the mammalian prion protein (PrP) is at the root of the fatal neurodegenerative disease transmissible spongiform encephalopathies (TSE), which afflicts humans, cattle, sheep, deer, and other animals. Prions have also been implicated in Alzheimer's disease. There have been intense efforts to develop therapies for TSE, based on chemotherapeutics and antibodies, that would act by modulating the expression and stability of PrP, although it remains unclear whether the soluble, properly folded form of PrP has important functions in the cell. Despite decades of research on the severity of prion-mediated disease in mammals, beneficial roles for the prion form of some proteins have recently been coming into view. The irreversible aggregation of proteins effectively results in robust amplification of immune signaling. There is also evidence that prions could be important for the formation of immune memory. Two examples of mammalian proteins that could be functional in their prion form are MAVS and ASC. MAVS aggregates in response to the highly sensitive binding of the RIG-I protein to viral RNA inside the cell. Following binding, RIG-I oligomerizes and activates

MAVS, which in turn leads to the induction of antiviral cytokine expression. Several experimental findings first suggested that MAVS forms prions: the protein gathers into complexes that are resistant to treatment with 2% sodium dodecyl sulfate (SDS), and the addition of these complexes to recombinant MAVS proteins in vitro caused these proteins to form protease-resistant cores. Furthermore, the MAVS prion state can be propagated through cell divisions. Nevertheless MAVS does stand apart from other typical prions in several ways. For one, their polymerization leads to gain of function. In addition, their polymerization is not stochastic but in response to activation by upstream sensors. Still, the other prion-like qualities of MAVS qualify it to be in this group of proteins. Once MAVS is activated by RIG-I, it forms punctate structures in the cell that are thought to be important for recruiting other proteins that help propagate its signal. Although MAVS is one of the first gain-of-function prions to be described in mammalian cells, there is evidence that these types of proteins are evolutionarily conserved. For example, when the fungal protein HET-S protein converts from soluble to aggregated, it can signal cell death to surrounding cells that do not contain HET-S prions. This finding suggests that prion state could possibly act as a form of memory for the cell of previous infection or insult. There is speculation that mammalian prions could serve a similar function and help explain the mechanism whereby mammalian cells are desensitized to pathogen stimulation and other threats.

39. Which of the following would be expected to diminish the levels of prions?
   a. Boiling
   b. Cell division
   c. Incineration
   d. Treatment with 2% SDS

40. Which of the following properties would be a benefit of using anti-PrP antibodies to treat prion disease?
   a. Immune tolerance
   b. Ability to distinguish aggregated from soluble PrP
   c. Ability to suppress expression of the PrP gene
   d. Poor transport across the blood-brain barrier

41. In what way are prions and microtubules similar to each other?
   a. Their polymerization is reversible.
   b. They are cytoplasmically inherited.
   c. They are not functional in their soluble form.
   d. Polymerization is associated with conformational change.

42. How many molecules of ATP are produced by the oxidation of one molecule of glucose?
   a. 8
   b. 16
   c. 32
   d. 64

43. Acute pancreatitis is caused by the inability of the pancreas to secrete which type of molecule?
   a. Bicarbonate
   b. Glucose
   c. Lipids
   d. Zymogens

44. Which of the following reactions would NOT be expected to occur spontaneously?

　　a. H_2O (*l*) → H_2O (*g*) (when the partial pressure of water vapor in the air < 0.031 atm)

　　b. $3O_2$ (*g*) → $2O_3$ (*g*)

　　c. CH_4 (*g*) + $2O_2$ (*g*) → CO_2 (*g*) + $2H_2O$ (*l*)

　　d. $2H_2$ (*g*) + O_2 (*g*) → $2H_2O$ (*g*)

45. Which of the following changes would explain a shift in the absorption spectra of a flavoprotein from 450 nm to 360 nm?

　　a. The flavoprotein changed from partially oxidized to fully oxidized.

　　b. The flavoprotein changed from fully oxidized to partially oxidized.

　　c. The flavoprotein changed from partially reduced to fully reduced.

　　d. The flavoprotein changed from fully reduced to partially reduced.

46. How many acetyl-CoA molecules does the fatty acid oxidation of palmitic acid $(C1_6H_{32}O_2)$ yield?

　　a. 4

　　b. 8

　　c. 16

　　d. 20

Use the following images to answer questions 47 and 48.

The following chemical structures represent progesterone (left) and testosterone (right).

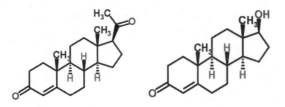

47. Based on these chemical structures, what is the single difference between the two steroid hormones?

　　a. Progesterone has a ketone; testosterone has an alcohol.

　　b. Progesterone has an alcohol; testosterone has a ketone.

　　c. Progesterone has an aldehyde; testosterone has an alcohol.

　　d. Progesterone has an alcohol; testosterone has an aldehyde.

48. In what conformation are the methyl and hydrogen groups in the A/B rings of these hormones?

　　a. cis-cis-cis

　　b. cis-trans-cis

　　c. trans-cis-trans

　　d. trans-trans-trans

49. Calculate the osmotic pressure of a 0.035-molar solution of nitrous acid at 295 Kelvin, given that the Van 't Hoff factor of nitrous acid is 1.1 and the gas constant is 0.08206 L atm mol^{-1} K^{-1}.

　　a. 0.63

　　b. 0.77

　　c. 0.85

　　d. 0.93

50. Which of the following is NOT an oncogenic cell surface receptor?

　　a. EGFR

　　b. ERBB2

　　c. TIM22

　　d. VEGF

51. The first step in the biosynthesis of terpenoids is the conversion of isopentenyl diphosphate (IPP) to dimethylallyl diphosphate (DMAPP), as depicted below. Which type of reaction is this conversion?

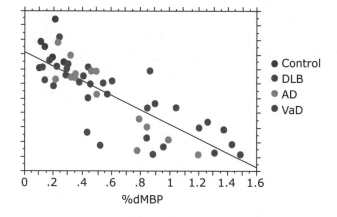

http://openi.nlm.nih.gov/detailedresult.php?img=2849937_401_
2009_635_Fig4_HTML&query=myelin%20sheath&it=xg&req=4
&npos=100.

   a. Isomerization
   b. Phosphorylation
   c. Condensation
   d. Reduction

Use the following information to answer questions 52 and 53.

The following graph displays the results of a study of post-mortem brain tissue from individuals with dementia with Lewy bodies (DLB), Alzheimer's disease (AD), vascular dementia (VaD), and health controls. Tissue sections were immunostained for degraded myelin basic protein (dMBP).

52. Based on the graph, which disease is associated with the most extensive myelin degeneration?
   a. Dementia with Lewy bodies
   b. Alzheimer's
   c. Vascular dementia
   d. They are associated with similar amounts of myelin degeneration.

53. Which type of molecule is used for immunostaining?
   a. Antibody
   b. ICAM
   c. MHC
   d. Synthetic chemical

54. What is the force that it would take for a molecule of sodium to spontaneously go through an ion channel in frog muscle? The concentration of Na+ inside and outside of muscle cells is 10.4 mM and 109 mM, respectively; the temperature is 285 Kelvin; and the V_m, or resting membrane potential, is −60 mV. The gas constant and Faraday constant are 8.31 joules/mol·K and 9.65×10^4 coulombs/ mol, respectively.
   a. 4.9×10^6
   b. 5.8×10^6
   c. 1.71×10^9
   d. 3.22×10^{10}

55. Which of the following changes results in membrane repolarization following the action potential of a neuron?
   a. Efflux of K^+
   b. Action of the ATP-dependent Na-K pump
   c. Influx of Cl^- passively into the neuron
   d. Opening of Na^+ channels

56. Which of the following properties do the endocrine system and neurons have in common?
   a. They primarily transmit messages through paracrine signaling.
   b. They transmit their signals (hormones and neurotransmitters) primarily via the bloodstream.
   c. They can transmit specific messages using the same type of hormone or neurotransmitter molecule.
   d. They respond to extracellular calcium through exocytosis.

57. How are cortical and trabecular bones similar to each other?

  a. They have similar rates of turnover.

  b. They have the same type of microstructure.

  c. They are made up of the same mineral components.

  d. They are similarly affected by osteoporotic fractures.

58. Which of the following statements about the digestive system is NOT true?

  a. Digestion starts in the mouth.

  b. Muscle contractions called peristalsis move food through the esophagus and intestines.

  c. Passing stool occurs when the sphincters relax and the rectum contracts.

  d. The main function of the liver is to detoxify chemicals that could be harmful.

59. Which of the following pathways directs the differentiation of multipotent skin cells into hair follicles?

  a. Hippo

  b. Notch

  c. Ras/Raf/MAP kinase

  d. Wnt/Wingless

Part 2: Chemical and Physical Foundations of Biological Systems

95 Minutes

59 Questions

1. As an ambulance with a blaring siren approaches, the pitch (frequency) of the sound

  a. increases, per the Doppler effect.

  b. decreases, per the Doppler effect.

  c. increases, per the Venturi effect.

  d. decreases, per the Venturi effect.

2. A box of mass 500 kg is pulled on a wagon across a level floor. A man pulls the wagon handle horizontally at a 50 degree angle by exerting a force of 240 N. The force of friction is 100 N. What is the acceleration of the wagon?

  a. 10.8 cm/s^2

  b. 16.8 cm/s^2

  c. 50.8 cm/s^2

  d. 56.8 cm/s^2

3. The least-stable non-planar conformation for a cyclic hexose carbohydrate is the

  a. boat conformation.

  b. chair conformation.

  c. half-chair conformation.

  d. twist-boat conformation.

4. The number of proton nuclear magnetic resonance (NMR) signals produced by 2-methylfluorobenzene is

  a. 1.

  b. 3.

  c. 5.

  d. 7.

5. A 1.0-kg sugar cube ($C_{12}H_{22}O_{11}$) is dissolved in 400 mL of acetone (density = 0.791 g/mL). What is the molality of the sugar solution?

  a. 7.3 mol/L

  b. 7.3 mol/kg

  c. 9.2 mol/L

  d. 9.2 mol/kg

Use the following information to answer questions 6 through 9.

Cyclodextrins (CDs) are a group of naturally cyclic oligosaccharides consisting of six, seven, or eight glucose subunits connected by α-(1,4) glycosidic bonds, named α-, β-, and γ-CDs, respectively. They are shaped cylindrically, with glycosidic oxygen bridges on the inside and hydroxyl groups on the outside. CDs can form inclusion complexes with molecules whose moieties interact with their internal surfaces. A novel method was developed for the preparation of β-CD functionalized magnetic nanoparticles (MNPs) (Figure 1).

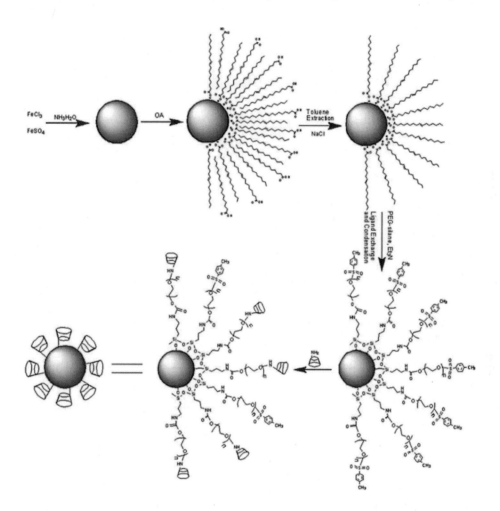

Figure 1. The preparation of β-CD functionalized magnetic nanoparticles. After OA-coated MNP synthesis, monotosyl-PEG silane was immobilized on them, and then toluene washes removed residual monotosyl-PEG silane and displaced OA. The material was dried in a vacuum, and then the MNPs were dispersed into DMF.

Monotosyl-polyethylene glycol (PEG) silane was synthesized by the route shown in Figure 2, where a PEG diol was modified to form the corresponding monotosyl-PEG, followed by reaction of the molecule with IPTS. ^{1}H NMR and FTIR spectroscopy were used to track molecule formation after each step, ultimately confirming formation of monotosyl-PEG silane. The nanoparticles were modified with the monotosyl-PEG silane first, and then amino-β-CD units displaced the tosyl units.

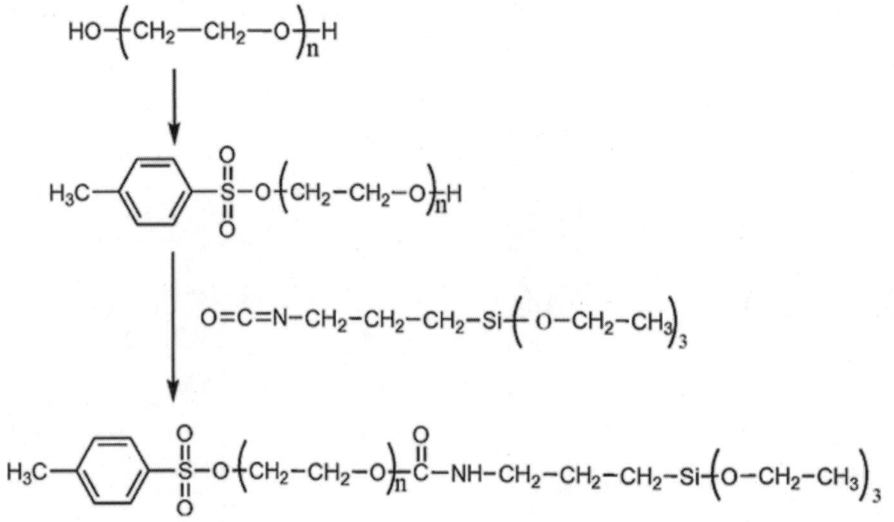

Figure 2. Preparation of monotosyl-PEG silane.
Y. Wu et al. A novel approach to molecular recognition surface of magnetic nanoparticles based on host-guest effect. *Nanoscale Res Lett.* 2009;4:738–747.

6. Moieties that are most likely to interact with CDs in inclusion complexes are
   a. positively charged.
   b. negatively charged.
   c. hydrophobic.
   d. amphipathic.

7. The first reaction step in Figure 2 can be completed by reacting PEG, tosyl chloride, and
   a. a weak acid in an S_N1 reaction.
   b. a weak base in an S_N1 reaction.
   c. a weak acid in an S_N2 reaction.
   d. a weak base in an S_N2 reaction.

8. The reason for the inclusion of tosyl groups in the synthesis is to
   a. contribute an oxygen to the functionalized final product.
   b. contribute a sulfur to the functionalized product.
   c. provide an effective leaving group for the ensuing nucleophilic attack.
   d. promote reactivity at the adjacent oxygen originally on the PEG diol.

9. Which intermediate or product in this synthesis does the FTIR spectrum below represent?

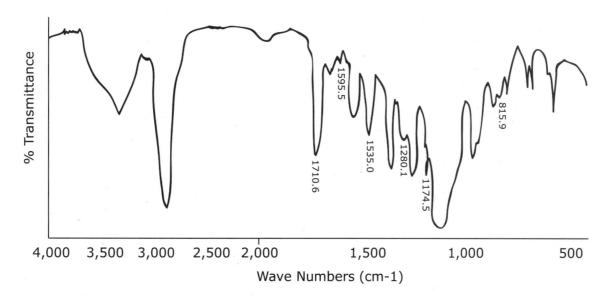

a. PEG diol
b. OA-MNPs
c. monotosyl-PEG silane
d. β-CD–PEG–MNPs

Use the following information to answer questions 10 through 14.

Indoleamine 2,3-dioxygenase (IDO) 1 catalyzes the first and rate-limiting step of L-tryptophan degradation in the tryptophan-kynurenine pathway. The direct product of IDO1 is N′-formylkynurenine, which breaks down non-enzymatically to L-kynurenine by losing its formyl group.

His-tagged human IDO1 cDNA was expressed in *Escherichia coli* and purified using a nickel column. IDO1 activity was measured in the absence and presence of various potential inhibitors in buffer at pH 6.5. Galanal was found to inhibit IDO1 activity, and based on the Michaelis-Menten kinetics of IDO1, its inhibitory mode was further studied by measuring the initial rate of L-kynurenine production in the presence and absence of 30 μM galanal at various L-tryptophan concentrations (Figure 1).

A

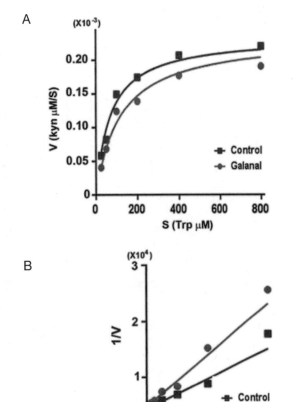

B

Figure 1. The effect of galanal on IDO1 activity.
R. Yamamoto et al. Effects of various phytochemicals on indole-amine 2,3-dioxygenase 1 activity: galanal is a novel, competitive inhibitor of the enzyme. *PLoS ONE.* 2014;9(2):e88789.

10. Based on the described enzymatic activity of IDO1, what is the structure of L-kynurenine?

a.

b.

c.

d.

11. The mode of IDO1 protein purification described in the passage is an example of
  a. size exclusion chromatography.
  b. affinity chromatography.
  c. anion exchange chromatography.
  d. cation exchange chromatography.

12. The following table provides pK_a values for four buffers at room temperature:

BUFFER	pK_a
Potassium phosphate	2.15, 7.20, 12.15
Potassium acetate	4.76
Tris	8.08
TEA	10.72

Which buffer would be most appropriate for measuring IPO1 reactivity?

a. Potassium phosphate

b. Potassium acetate

c. Tris

d. TEA

13. The graph used to study galanal inhibition of IDO1 in Figure 1B is called a(n)
a. Eadie-Hofstee diagram.
b. Lineweaver-Burk plot.
c. Hanes-Woolf plot.
d. Hill plot.

14. The mode of IDO1 inhibition by galanal is
a. competitive.
b. uncompetitive.
c. noncompetitive.
d. irreversible covalent adduct formation.

Use the following information to answer questions 15 through 19.

Myelin is an essential electrically insulating material that forms a layer around the axon of a neuron. The production of this myelin sheath is called myelination, and it begins in humans several months into fetal development. Although myelin is approximately 40% water, its dry mass is approximately 70% to 85% lipid and approximately 15% to 30% protein mass. The main lipid found in myelin is galactocerebroside, which can also be sulfated at carbon 3 on the galactose ring by sulphotransferase (Figure 1). The primary function of the myelin sheath is to increase the speed at which impulses propagate along the myelinated fiber, decreasing capacitance and increasing electrical resistance across the cell membrane. Impulses move continuously as waves along unmyelinated fibers, but saltatory conduction occurs along myelinated fibers, with intracellular and extracellular fluid separated strongly. The nodes of Ranvier, unlike the myelin sheath, contain many voltage-gated sodium channels that allow enough sodium into the axon to create an action potential. Diseases like multiple sclerosis and Guillain-Barré disease are caused by the destruction of the myelin sheath.

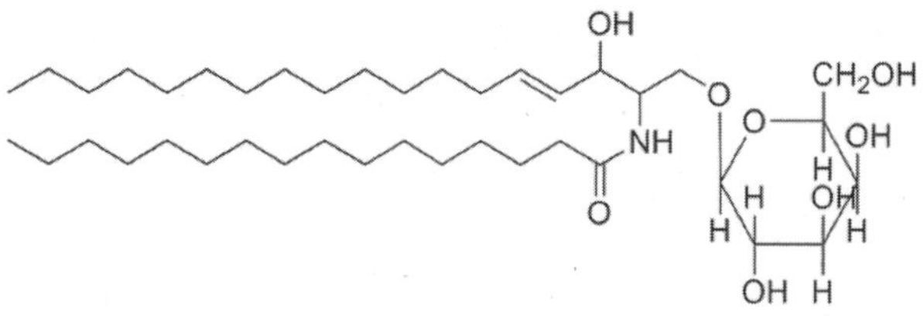

Figure 1. The structure of galactocerebroside.

15. The cells that produce the myelin sheath are called
a. Schwann cells.
b. presynaptic cells.
c. postsynaptic cells.
d. Langerhans cells.

16. Based on the structure in Figure 1, galactocerebroside is best categorized as a
a. sterol lipid.
b. glycerolipid.
c. fatty acid.
d. sphingolipid.

17. Based on the structure of galactocerebroside, the most stable configuration of the sulfated hydroxyl group in sulfated galactocerebroside is
   a. axial.
   b. equatorial.
   c. either axial or equatorial because both are equally stable.
   d. neither axial nor equatorial because the ring is a benzene ring, not a cyclohexose.

18. The myelin sheath helps to reduce energy expenditure over the overall axon membrane because
   a. it increases the permeability of the axon surface for transfer of sodium and potassium ions via diffusion, reducing the need for an ATP-requiring pump.
   b. it decreases the number of sodium and potassium ions that need to be pumped to restore resting state concentrations after each action potential.
   c. the increased impulse speed reduces the amount of work required for its propulsion through the axon, reducing the amount of ATP needed to do so.
   d. it decreases the pressure of the axon to increase the speed of the impulse through the axon.

19. Based on its functional description in the passage, myelin can be classified as a
   a. semiconductor.
   b. cathode.
   c. dielectric.
   d. refrigerant.

Use the following information to answer questions 20 through 23.

A woman of mass 55 kg begins motionless atop a hill. She skis all the way down the frictionless hill, which is 90 m high, to height 0 m, and then she ascends another hill that is 75 m high. This skier is in a conservative system, with gravity as the only force acting upon her.

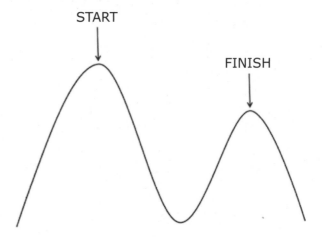

Figure 1. A diagram of the ski slopes.

20. In a conservative system like the one described in the passage, which of the following statements are true?

I. The work done by a force is completely reversible.
II. The work done by a force is dependent on the path taken.
III. The work done by a force is equal to the difference between the final and initial values of an energy function.

   a. I only
   b. I and II only
   c. I and III only
   d. I, II, and III

21. At what speed is the skier moving when she reaches the peak of the second hill?

a. 12.1 m/s

b. 17.1 m/s

c. 22.3 m/s

d. 25.0 m/s

22. How much of the skier's original potential energy is lost during her journey from the peak of the first hill to the peak of the second hill?

a. 1.24 kJ

b. 2.45 kJ

c. 5.76 kJ

d. 8.09 kJ

23. At which point in her ski route will the skier have the greatest amount of kinetic energy?

a. At the top of the first hill

b. Halfway down the first hill

c. At a height of 0 m between the hills

d. Halfway up the second hill

Use the following information to answer questions 24 through 31.

The Bradford assay is a common analytical technique that is used to measure the concentration of protein in a solution. It is both a spectroscopic and colorimetric procedure that is based on the absorbance shift of the Coomassie Brilliant Blue G-250 dye (Figure 1). The dye exists in the three forms: cationic (red), neutral (green), and anionic (blue). Under the acidic conditions used to perform the assay, the red form of the dye binds the protein and is converted to a stable blue anionic form, disrupting the native state of the protein and exposing its hydrophobic pockets. The hydrophobic regions of the protein bind to the nonpolar region of the dye, and the amine groups of the protein are placed near the negatively charged substituents on the dye. When protein binds the dye, the complex is stabilized and exhibits an absorbance maximum at 595 nm that is proportional to the amount of bound dye.

Though the Bradford assay is less susceptible to interference by other chemicals that might be present in the protein solution, the presence of the organic anionic detergent sodium dodecyl sulfate (SDS) can disrupt the Bradford assay, working by two different modes at low and high concentrations to impact the absorbance readings at 595 nm.

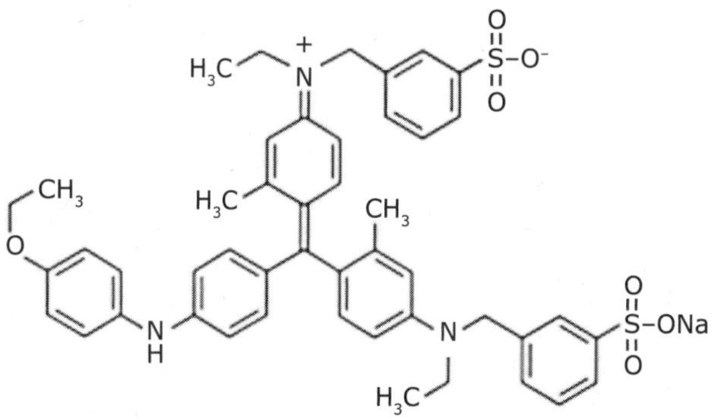

Figure 1. The structure of Coomassie Brilliant Blue G-250 dye in its green form.

24. Which amino acid might accept a proton from the dye?

a. Arginine

b. Glutamic acid

c. Cysteine

d. Glutamine

25. According to the passage, the intermolecular forces that are most essential for stabilizing the complex between the dye and the unfolded protein are

I. hydrogen bonds
II. van der Waals forces
III. ionic forces

a. I and II only
b. I and III only
c. II and III only
d. I, II, and III

26. The absorbance of a newly discovered protein at 595 nm is determined, normalized with the appropriate baseline spectrum. If the protein concentration is to be directly calculated from this absorbance, what additional information is needed?
a. The molecular weight of the protein, determined via size-exclusion chromatography using a set of molecular weight standards
b. The dissociation constant for the binding of the dye to the protein of interest
c. The spectrum for the red form of the dye for A_{595} correction
d. The equation of the standard curve line relating A_{595} and a series of known concentrations of a standard protein

27. The Beer-Lambert law relates light absorption to the properties of the material of interest through the equation $A = \varepsilon bc$, where A is absorbance in the Bradford assay, ε is the molar absorptivity (L mol^{-1} cm^{-1}) of the material, b is the path length of the cuvette containing the sample in the spectrometer, and c is the concentration (mol/L) of the material in solution. If one wishes to determine the molar absorptivity of a particular protein, it is absolutely essential that
a. all cofactors have been removed from the protein.
b. the protein is in its correct polymeric form.
c. the protein is extremely pure.
d. there are tryptophan residues in the protein.

28. Why might SDS be present in a purified protein solution immediately following a standard purification procedure?
a. SDS is commonly used to support cellular growth in growth media.
b. SDS is used for protein separation in SDS-PAGE.
c. SDS is commonly used to lyse cells by disrupting the membrane lipid bilayer.
d. Most methods of column chromatography require the use of SDS for resin stabilization.

29. How might SDS interact with the dye to disrupt the Bradford assay?
a. SDS associates strongly with the red and green forms of the dye, increasing the absorbance at 595 nm independently of protein presence.
b. SDS associates strongly with the red and green forms of the dye, decreasing the absorbance at 595 nm independently of protein presence.
c. SDS associates strongly with the blue form of the dye, increasing the absorbance at 595 nm independently of protein presence.
d. SDS associates strongly with the blue form of the dye, decreasing the absorbance at 595 nm independently of protein presence.

30. How might SDS interact with the protein to disrupt the Bradford assay?

    a. SDS binds to the protein, blocking protein binding sites for the dye and causing overestimation of the protein concentration.

    b. SDS binds to the protein, blocking protein binding sites for the dye and causing underestimation of the protein concentration.

    c. SDS binds to the protein, enhancing protein-dye interactions and causing overestimation of the protein concentration.

    d. SDS binds to the protein, enhancing protein-dye interactions and causing underestimation of the protein concentration.

31. The passage provides the wavelength of maximum absorbance for the blue form of the dye. Based on the electromagnetic spectrum and principles of light absorption, the wavelengths of maximum absorbance for the red and green forms, respectively, are

    a. 250 nm and 470 nm.

    b. 470 nm and 250 nm.

    c. 470 nm and 650 nm.

    d. 650 nm and 470 nm.

32. A round hole with a diameter of 10 cm is cut into a sheet of brass. The coefficient of linear thermal expansion (α) is $18.9 \times 10^{-6} \div °C$. What will be the change in area of the hole when the temperature is increased by 50°C?

    a. $0.00 \ cm^2$

    b. $7.40 \times 10^{-2} \ cm^2$

    c. $0.148 \ cm^2$

    d. $0.594 \ cm^2$

33. Xylem is a transport tissue found in vascular plants that transports water and nutrients. A xylem tube pushes xylem sap upward through the plant via capillary action. Which of the following principles is NOT responsible for this phenomenon?

    a. Surface tension

    b. Buoyancy

    c. Cohesion

    d. Adhesion

34. A proton travels at 7.5×10^7 m/s perpendicularly to a magnetic field that causes it to move in a circular path with a 1.00 m radius. The mass of a proton is 1.67×10^{-27} kg, and the charge of a proton is 1.60×10^{-19} c. What is the strength of the magnetic field?

    a. 0.139 T

    b. 0.783 T

    c. 1.28 T

    d. 7.19 T

35. Lead chloride dissolves, to a limited extent, in water by the following equilibrium expression:

$$PbCl_2(s) \rightleftharpoons Pb^{2+}(aq) + 2Cl^-(aq)$$

How does the addition of NaCl to the solution affect $PbCl_2$ solubility and the K_{sp}?

    a. $PbCl_2$ solubility increases and K_{sp} decreases.

    b. $PbCl_2$ solubility increases and K_{sp} stays the same.

    c. $PbCl_2$ solubility decreases and K_{sp} decreases.

    d. $PbCl_2$ solubility decreases and K_{sp} stays the same.

36. In Ernest Rutherford's famous gold foil experiment, Rutherford studied the angles of radiation particle scattering as the particles passed through a thin sheet of gold foil. Most particles passed through without deflection, but a few particles were deflected at various angles. The scattering was attributed to repulsion of the particles by the atomic nuclei in the foil. The type of radiation particles Rutherford used, therefore, were

   a. neutrons.

   b. α particles.

   c. β particles.

   d. γ particles.

37. The fourth ionization energy of aluminum is immensely higher than the first three ionization energies because

   a. a significant amount of energy is needed to remove an electron from the filled-shell configuration of the Al^{3+} ion.

   b. the force of repulsion between the electron being added and the electrons already present is significantly higher.

   c. the first three ionization energies do not require electron excitation, but this requirement greatly increases the fourth ionization energy.

   d. the mass of the Al^{3+} ion increases significantly during this transition, and energy is inversely proportional to mass.

38. A 250-g calorimeter with a specific heat capacity of 20.0 J/g · °C contains 600 g of water (c = 4.18 J/g · °C). Given that the molar heat of combustion of sucrose, $C_{12}H_{22}O_{11}$, releases 5.65×10^3 kJ of heat, what mass of sucrose must be burned to increase the temperature of the water *and* calorimeter by 10°C?

   a. 1.52 g

   b. 3.03 g

   c. 4.55 g

   d. 7.90 g

39. Purified ATPase was incubated with 200 μM dicyclohexylcarbodiimide (DCCD) at pH 7.6 (A) and 9.0 (B). Individual mixtures contained no NaCl (open circles), 1 mM NaCl (closed triangles), 10 mM NaCl (open triangles), and 50 mM NaCl (closed squares). ATPase reactivity was initiated by 4 mM ATP, and the residual ATPase activity of the samples was measured at various times. The graph with the closed circles is the control with no DCCD.

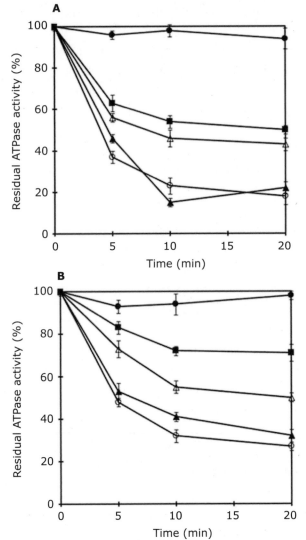

Image from A. Soontharapirakkul and K. Incharoensakdi. Na+-stimulated ATPase of alkaliphilic halo-tolerant cyanobacterium *Aphanothece halophytica* translocates Na+ into proteoliposomes via Na+ uniport mechanism. *BMC Biochemistry*. 2010;11:30.

Which of the conclusions about the role of Na⁺ in the activity of this ATPase is valid based on the collected data?

a. Na⁺ effectively inhibits ATPase activity, but its inhibition is weakened in the presence of DCCD.
b. Increasing concentration of Na⁺ effectively protects against DCCD inhibition of the ATPase.
c. Na⁺ and DCCD work together in a cooperative fashion to inhibit the activity of this ATPase.
d. Na⁺ and DCCD work together in a cooperative fashion to stimulate the activity of this ATPase.

40. According to Faraday's laws of electrolysis, the masses of substances formed during electrolysis at an electrode are
a. directly proportional to the quantity of electricity that passes through the electrolyte.
b. inversely proportional to the quantity of electricity that passes through the electrolyte.
c. directly proportional to the capacitance of the system.
d. inversely proportional to the capacitance of the system.

41. When ice is placed in a vessel and heated at 55°C, it melts. Which of the following statements are true?
   I. The change in free energy is positive.
   II. The change in entropy is positive.
   III. The change in enthalpy is positive.
a. I and II only
b. I and III only
c. II and III only
d. I, II, and III

42. The van der Waals equation modifies the ideal gas law to account for deviations of real gases from ideal gas behavior. The two factors the equation takes into consideration are
a. phase changes and chemical bonding.
b. molecular expansion and chemical transformations.
c. molecular volume and molecular attractions.
d. molecular masses and partial pressures.

Use the following information to answer questions 43 through 46.

A scientist accidentally mixed together concentrated pure samples of four well-characterized human proteins. The proteins were diluted into buffer of pH 6.0. The following table provides general data about the four proteins:

PROTEIN	MOLECULAR WEIGHT (kDa)	pI	FUNCTION
Calmodulin I	16.7	3.9	Binds Ca^{2+} and transduces calcium signals
Glucokinase	50.9	5.0	Phosphorylates glucose to glucose-6-phosphate using ATP
Hemoglobin	16.0	6.9	Binds and transports oxygen
Transferrin (diferric)	80.0	5.2	Binds and transports iron

The scientist first separated the proteins based on molecular weight, which allowed for the isolation of glucokinase and transferrin because their molecular weights were distinct. The buffer was exchanged in the solution containing the other two proteins, replacing the pH 6.0 buffer with pH 5.0 buffer. The scientist then used the difference in pI to separate calmodulin I and hemoglobin by anion exchange chromatography, as the molecular weights of these proteins were too close to separate by the previous method without time-consuming optimization.

After obtaining pure samples of the four proteins through this purification strategy, the scientist added appropriate cofactors to the proteins, took UV-visible spectra of each protein, and then tested the binding of several molecules to each protein in order to confirm the appropriate identities of the four proteins. The UV-visible spectrum of hemoglobin notably included a large Soret peak around 412 nm, and this sample was successfully able to bind oxygen.

43. A possible method by which the scientist could have isolated glucokinase and transferrin during the protocol described in the passage is
   a. paper chromatography.
   b. SDS-PAGE.
   c. distillation.
   d. gel filtration chromatography.

44. Which technique would be suitable to use for buffer exchange between the two separation methods, as described in the passage?
   a. Dialysis
   b. Affinity chromatography
   c. High-pressure liquid chromatography
   d. Extraction

45. When the solution of calmodulin I and hemoglobin is separated during the second purification step, which protein(s) will bind the resin?
   a. Hemoglobin only
   b. Calmodulin I only
   c. Both hemoglobin and calmodulin I
   d. Neither hemoglobin nor calmodulin I

46. The observed Soret peak in the hemoglobin UV-visible spectrum, as described in the passage, is caused by
   a. α-helices in the active site pocket.
   b. β-sheets in the active site pocket.
   c. the tryptophan residues in the protein.
   d. the π electrons in the bound porphyrin ring.

Use the following information to answer questions 47 through 51.

The reaction of gaseous carbon dioxide and steam results in the formation of oxygen gas and acetylene gas. A balanced equation for this reaction is shown below:

$$4CO_2(g) + 2H_2O(g) \rightarrow 2C_2H_2(g) + 5O_2(g)$$

ΔH values are provided for a series of related reactions:

$$C_2H_2(g) + 2H_2(g) \rightarrow C_2H_6(g) \qquad \Delta H = -94.5 \text{ kJ}$$

$$H_2O(g) \rightarrow H_2(g) + \tfrac{1}{2}O_2(g) \qquad \Delta H = -71.2 \text{ kJ}$$

$$C_2H_6(g) + \tfrac{7}{2}O_2(g) \rightarrow 2CO_2(g) + 3H_2O(g)$$
$$\Delta H = -283 \text{ kJ}$$

47. What is the value of ΔH for the overall reaction of carbon dioxide with steam?
   a. -306 kJ
   b. $+235$ kJ
   c. $+306$ kJ
   d. $+470$ kJ

48. If 2.0 g each of $CO_2(g)$ and $H_2O(g)$ react completely, what mass of C_2H_2 will be produced?

    a. 0.59 g

    b. 1.2 g

    c. 2.4 g

    d. 2.9 g

49. The value of ΔS for the reaction of $CO_2(g)$ and $H_2O(g)$ is

    a. positive because a greater number of moles of CO_2 than H_2O are required for the reaction.

    a. negative because a greater number of moles of CO_2 than H_2O are required for the reaction.

    c. positive because the number of gas molecules increases over the course of the reaction.

    d. negative because the number of gas molecules increases over the course of the reaction.

50. When $CO_2(g)$ and $H_2O(g)$ react, the two gaseous products are collected in separate containers. If 5.00 g CO_2 reacts with an excess of H_2O, what volume of O_2 will be produced at STP (standard temperature and pressure), given that the ideal gas constant, R, is equal to $0.08206 \frac{L \cdot atm}{mol \cdot K}$?

    a. 0.373 L

    b. 1.27 L

    c. 2.55 L

    d. 3.18 L

51. The VSEPR shape of $CO_2(g)$ is

    a. bent.

    b. tetrahedral.

    c. T-shaped.

    d. linear.

Use the following information to answer questions 52 through 55.

Nickel (II) oxide (NiO) is often deposited as a thin film onto glass substrates through spray pyrolysis. The electrical properties of the NiO film were characterized experimentally. The electrical resistivity was recorded within the approximate 30°C to 170°C range (Figure 1). In addition, the activation energy of conductivity was determined by plotting the natural log of the DC conductivity as a function of $1000/T$ (Figure 2). The NiO film was also, importantly, characterized structurally using X-ray diffraction.

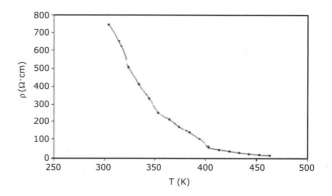

Figure 1. Resistivity as a function of temperature for NiO films.

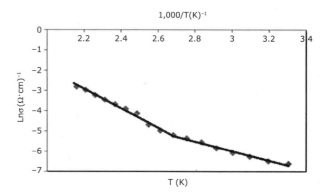

Figure 2. Activation energy for NiO films.

A. Hassan. Study of optical and electrical properties of nickel oxide (NiO) thin films deposited by using a spray pyrolysis technique. *J Modern Phys.* 2014;5:2184–2191.

52. The key difference between resistance and resistivity is that
    a. resistance is a state function, whereas resistivity is not.
    b. resistance is dependent on sample dimensions, whereas resistivity is not.
    c. resistivity is temperature dependent, whereas resistance is not.
    d. resistance is the product of the Boltzmann constant and the resistivity.

53. The structural characterization technique described in the passage provides information about
    a. the susceptibility of the NiO film to oxidation or reduction.
    b. the NiO film's crystalline phase and unit cell dimensions.
    c. the presence of excited electrons in the NiO film.
    d. the Ni-O bond lengths and bond angles.

54. The electrical data collected in Figures 1 and 2 support the conclusion that
    a. NiO films are conductors.
    b. NiO films are magnets.
    c. NiO films are insulators.
    d. NiO films are semiconductors.

55. The activation energy can be determined using the data in Figure 2 by multiplying the Boltzmann constant by
    a. the slope of each line, at high and low temperatures.
    b. the y-intercept of each line, at high and low temperatures.
    c. the x-intercept of each line, at high and low temperatures.
    d. the sum of the y-intercept and the x-intercept of each line, at high and low temperatures.

Use the following information to answer questions 56 through 59.

The structure of adenosine triphosphate (ATP) is shown below (Figure 1). ATP is hydrolyzed to ADP and inorganic phosphate when in equilibrium with water, and the high energy of this molecule comes from two high-energy phosphoanhydride bonds. Each bond has a ΔG of -30.5 kJ/mol. Therefore, the free energy released by hydrolysis of ATP to ADP and inorganic phosphate under standard conditions, $\Delta G^{\circ\prime}$, is equal to -30.5 kJ/mol at pH 7.0.

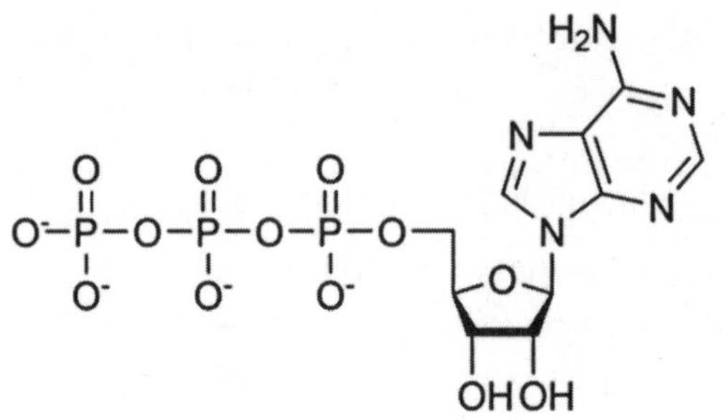

Figure 1. The structure of ATP.

56. The nucleoside component of ATP is a
    a. porphyrin.
    b. purine.
    c. pyrimidine.
    d. flavin.

57. The value for $\Delta G^{\circ\prime}$ indicates that ATP hydrolysis is
    a. exothermic.
    b. endothermic.
    c. exergonic.
    d. endergonic.

58. The following table provides the concentrations of ATP, ADP, and P_i in human erythrocytes:

MOLECULE	CONCENTRATION IN HUMAN ERYTHROCYTES (mM)
ATP	2.24
ADP	0.25
P_i	1.65

Given that the constant R is equal to $0.08314 \frac{kJ}{mol \cdot K}$, and assuming equilibrium at pH 7.0 and body temperature of 37°C, what is the free energy of hydrolysis of ATP under these conditions?

a. −52 kJ/mol
b. −41 kJ/mol
c. −33 kJ/mol
d. −8.5 kJ/mol

59. The observed $\Delta G^{\circ\prime}$ for ATP hydrolysis to ADP and inorganic phosphate CANNOT be attributed to
a. electrostatic repulsions among the negative oxygen atoms in ATP.
b. greater resonance stabilization of ADP relative to ATP.
c. lower solvation of inorganic phosphate, H^+, and ADP relative to ATP.
d. higher disorder and lower free energy in ADP relative to ATP.

Part 3: Psychological, Social, and Biological Foundations of Behavior

59 Questions
95 Minutes

Use the following images to answer questions 1 through 5.

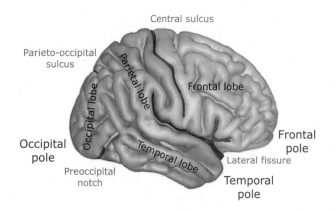

Human brain, image 1.
http://en.wikipedia.org/wiki/Central_sulcus#/media/File:LobesCaptsLateral.png.

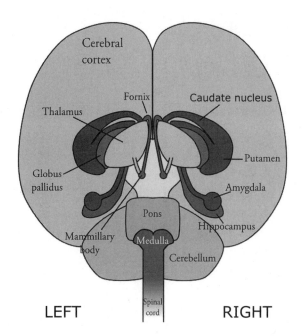

Human brain, image 2.
http://pixabay.com/en/brain-diagram-medical-biology-40356/.

1. A man becomes very angry with his neighbor for taking his parking spot. Which part of the brain evokes this emotion?
   a. Occipital pole
   b. Amygdala
   c. Cerebellum
   d. Fornix

2. Typically, people cope with stress with either emotion-focused or problem-focused strategies. If the man utilizes a problem-focused coping strategy, he could do any of the following EXCEPT
   a. approach the neighbor to see if there is a misunderstanding.
   b. speak with the apartment complex management about a possible alternate parking spot.
   c. write a letter to the apartment association about the need for strict parking guidelines.
   d. vent to other people about the problem.

3. Which lobe of the brain receives and processes sensory information from the body?
   a. Frontal
   b. Occipital
   c. Parietal
   d. Temporal

4. What do olfactory pathways do in the brain?
   a. Carry the sense of smell from the nose to the brain to be processed
   b. Carry visual images from the eyes to the brain to be processed
   c. Carry the tastes of food from the tongue to the brain to be processed
   d. Carry sounds from the ears to the brain to be processed

5. Brain damage in which lobe of the brain would MOST affect higher-level cognition?
   a. Frontal
   b. Occipital
   c. Parietal
   d. Temporal

Use the following passage to answer questions 6 through 10.

A graduate student is interested in changing her teaching from a traditional method to one that includes significantly more discourse with her students. She is a teaching assistant for a first-semester biology course at the same university where she is pursuing her master's level secondary (teaching) biology certification and degree. A study researcher is interested in documenting the graduate student's experience as she attempts to implement this new method.

The researcher videotapes the graduate student each week as she is teaching her class; the graduate student views the tape later while being interviewed about what happened both in the class and outside of the class. Surprisingly, the individuals who experience the most cognitive dissonance about the teaching methodology are not the students or the graduate student, but rather the graduate student's supervisors in the biology department. The new teaching method is the first of its kind, and limited success was expected. The student teacher decides to continue the new teaching method regardless of her supervisors' opinions. When the findings suggest the methodology to be beneficial, the supervisors have a change of mind and support the new methodology.

6. Which of the following is the BEST example of what cognitive dissonance may have looked like in this research study?

   a. The supervisors were confused and disapproved of the teaching method because it was different from how college biology is usually taught.

   b. The supervisors were pleased that the student teacher was trying an innovative teaching method and planned to implement it with other teachers.

   c. The supervisors received a lot of complaints from the students in the class and disciplined the student teacher for her new teaching method.

   d. The supervisors were initially happy with the new teaching method but grew tired of hearing complaints from other student teachers by the end of the study.

7. Which type of research methodology was performed in this study?

   a. Case study

   b. Experimental

   c. Split-half

   d. Item equating

8. What is the MOST likely expectation of the supervisors of the graduate student in this study?

   a. Peer pressure

   b. Conformity

   c. Role playing

   d. Social loafing

9. The graduate student's decision to continue implementing the new method instead of reverting to the more familiar, traditional method despite her supervisors' cognitive dissonance means she probably had a high level of

   a. self-fulfilling prophecy.

   b. stereotype threat.

   c. self-efficacy.

   d. stigma.

10. The supervisors were likely comparing the graduate student to which group?

   a. Class identity group

   b. Self-identity group

   c. Power group

   d. Reference group

11. An Internet phenomenon in 2015 featured a picture of a dress that different people saw as different colors. Some saw it as blue and black, while others saw it as white and gold. Which of the following is the BEST term for the process responsible for people forming different color perceptions?

   a. Somatosensation

   b. Optic nerve malfunction

   c. Parallel processing

   d. Auditory processing

12. The "fight or flight" experience is centered in which system in the body?

   a. Endocrine

   b. Lymphatic

   c. Integumentary

   d. Cardiovascular

13. According to sociocognitive theory, the development of prejudice in self-identity begins at a young age. For example, small children are likely to believe that girls are not good at sports and that boys get into trouble more often. At what age is this likely to start to turn around to a more positive viewpoint?

a. 4 to 6 years old
b. 5 to 7 years old
c. 8 to 9 years old
d. 10 to 11 years old

14. Typically, what is the MAIN difference between how Eastern and Western cultures value aging?

a. Eastern cultures tend to provide financial incentives to the elderly, whereas Western cultures do not.
b. Aging in Eastern cultures is socially constructed, whereas aging in Western cultures is personally constructed.
c. Eastern cultures tend to value age and wisdom, whereas Western cultures tend to value youth.
d. Some Eastern cultures consider putting an elderly family member in a nursing home to be an acceptable way to deal with overpopulation, whereas in the West, it is usually done for health reasons.

15. Environmental justice advocates frequently make the argument that minority populations disproportionally undertake or are subjected to environmentally hazardous activities because they have few economic alternatives and/or are not fully aware of the risks involved. Which of the following is the STRONGEST statement a person questioning this kind of environmental racism might make?

a. Minority populations don't care about environmental issues.
b. Environmental advocacy groups want to put big businesses out of business.

c. Environmental issues like global warming do not really exist and are just part of the liberal agenda.
d. Environmental issues historically have been less important to minority groups than more pressing socioeconomic issues.

Use the following passage to answer questions 16 through 20.

Symbolic interactionism is a sociology theory based on ways of understanding the workings of the world in relation to oneself. It emphasizes the language and symbols that give meaning to how people see themselves, the world, and the relationships between them. As people interact with the world, they often change the way they behave based on how they define those interactions. They spend time thinking about what to do next depending on how they believe others view them.

Social interactionists believe that communications and interactions form the reality each individual identifies with. People create these realities based on external interactions and perceptions; thus, each person's reality is unique. Reality, according to this belief, is socially constructed, or created by thoughts, conversations, and ideas. Individuals both create and shape society, and the change occurring is constant and ongoing. Social interactionists are interested in the patterns created by people's interactions and how an individual's reality shapes his or her daily existence.

To better understand how social interactionists view the world, let's consider a specific example. Imagine two men who have worked in the same department of the same company for many years. They have been rivals, both at times attempting to score a big promotion. One of the men (Colleague A) is resentful of the other (Colleague B) because he perceives Colleague B as pointing out his weaknesses in front of colleagues and making jokes about him when all of the employees are out for happy-hour drinks. Through such interactions, Colleague A develops a negative viewpoint of Colleague B. Events will also be symbolic to Colleague A, and the man subjectively misperceives them. For instance, Colleague B gets married and receives the promotion they had both been trying to acquire. He perceives Colleague B's good fortune as a fact that he always gets what he wants and that all the good things happen to him. However, later in the year, Colleague B is fired and comes to Colleague A for support. Colleague A then feels needed and is able to be helpful to Colleague B. He no longer sees Colleague B as a threat but rather as a friend.

Symbolic interactionists would look at the example above and note how one man's view of the other shaped his reality of the situation. Before his colleague lost his job, Colleague A held one version of reality in his mind. He symbolically saw his colleague as having an unfair advantage in the world. When the dynamic shifted and the man played a role of support to his colleague, the meaning he gave to his relationship with him changed. All of this is based on the social interactions that occur, the language used to communicate, and the symbolic meaning given to these events and thoughts.

16. The passage states that "reality, according to this belief, is socially constructed, or created by thoughts, conversations, and ideas." Which of the following technologies would MOST directly contribute to the social construction of reality?
a. Television
b. Facebook or other social media
c. Satellite radio
d. A computer server

17. The example of the relationship between Colleague A and Colleague B falls within which of the following theories?
a. Social cognitive theory
b. Vygotskyian theory
c. Social conflict theory
d. Rational choice theory

18. Which of the following concepts BEST describes the relationship between the two colleagues?
a. Deviance
b. Collective behavior
c. Agent of socialization
d. Social norms

19. The evolution of Colleague A's emotions during the passage is MOST likely due to which of the following?
a. The adaptive role of emotion
b. Universal emotions
c. Child versus adult emotions
d. Brain development

20. Which part of the brain is MOST involved in the emotions the colleagues are experiencing in the passage?
a. The cerebellum
b. The cerebral cortex
c. The brain stem
d. The limbic system

Use the following passage to answer questions 21 through 26.

Adult students' ideas about scientific phenomena are strongly held and resistant to change. In the 1980s, a group of science educators came up with a theory of "conceptual change" to explain how these resistant scientific concepts could be changed via science instruction. They called this process *accommodation*, based on an earlier theory of "equilibration." The reason scientific conceptions are so resistant to change is that when new science content is learned, the learner's brain changes the new content to fit what the learner already knows and believes about science content. However, the science educators proposed a four-part process as a model for instructors to use to change existing misconceptions held by the learners. This process includes making concepts intelligible, meaning they make sense to the learners. They must also be made plausible to the learner, meaning the new concepts are believable. They must also be fruitful, meaning that the new concepts can be used to understand future phenomena they experience, as well as future science concepts. And, finally, they must be dissatisfied with their existing misconceptions. The authors, however, stated that these are conditions for learning and that it is a piecemeal and gradual process. They stated that all four conditions must be present for a misconception to be changed. Science educators since then have used the theory to create and test new instructional models based on the four conditions for conceptual change.

21. The concepts of accommodation and equilibration were first developed by which researcher(s)?
    a. James-Lange
    b. Maslow
    c. Piaget
    d. Vygotsky

22. When the brain changes new knowledge to fit existing knowledge, what is this process called?
    a. Accommodation
    b. Assimilation
    c. Equilibration
    d. Stage progression

23. A team of science education researchers developed an instructional model based on the theory presented in the passage. They wanted to test its effectiveness, so they trained one high school physical science teacher on how to use the instructional model and selected another physical science teacher from the same school who was considered "exemplary" but did not use the conceptual change knowledge. The two teachers taught a unit on electricity. The students were pre- and post-tested on their knowledge of the unit content. Which of the following is the dependent variable in this study?
    a. The students who received the conceptual change instruction
    b. The type of instruction provided to each of the two groups of students
    c. The difference in students' scores between the pre- and post-tests
    d. The teacher who did NOT provide the conceptual change instruction

24. When learners are put through a process of having their misconceptions challenged, they frequently experience negative emotions, such as anger and frustration. According to the conceptual change model, this is a necessary component of the model. Which theory BEST supports this process?
    a. Cognitive dissonance theory
    b. Negative feedback systems
    c. Behaviorist theory
    d. Biopsychosocial approach

25. Which agent of socialization is MOST responsible for the resistance to change scientific misconceptions?
    a. The family
    b. The media
    c. The student's peers
    d. The educational system

26. Which of the following parts of the conceptual change model is MOST likely to effect attitude change?
   a. Intelligibility
   b. Plausibility
   c. Fruitfulness
   d. Dissatisfaction

27. Which of the following is an example of bottom-up processing?
   a. Understanding a paragraph with difficult handwriting by using context
   b. Understanding a situation using past experiences
   c. Identifying details of a stimulus using perceptional signals
   d. Understanding that a visual illusion is difficult using contextual clues

28. Breast development in boys during adolescence is typically unwanted in Western cultures. What causes unwanted breast development to occur?
   a. It is a response to rising estradiol levels.
   b. It is a response to increased testosterone compared to estradiol.
   c. It is caused by menarche.
   d. It is caused by increased myelinization in males compared to females.

29. Which of the following is the BEST example of a fundamental attribution error?
   a. Someone trips on a dog and the observer assumes he did not see the dog, which in fact was the case.
   b. Someone trips on a dog and the observer assumes he does not like the dog, when in fact he did not see the dog.
   c. Someone trips on a dog and assumes it is because he can never do anything right.
   d. Someone trips on a dog, and it is a self-fulfilling prophecy.

30. All of the following are examples of social institutions EXCEPT
   a. marriage.
   b. education.
   c. the Internet.
   d. government.

Use the following passage to answer questions 31 through 33.

Protein misfolding and subsequent aggregation have been proven to be the leading cause of most known dementias. Many dementias, in addition to neurodegeneration, show profound changes in behavior and thinking, i.e., psychiatric symptoms. On the basis of the observation that progressive myoclonic epilepsies and neurodegenerative diseases share some common features of neurodegeneration, autophagy may be a common impairment in these diseases. A similar line could be argued for some neuropsychiatric conditions, among them depression and schizophrenia. Existing and new therapies for these seemingly different diseases could be augmented with drugs used for neurodegenerative or neuropsychiatric diseases, respectively, some of which modulate or augment autophagy.

31. The passage states that "autophagy may be a common impairment in these diseases." Given that autophagy is a normal cell function, what might be the impairment in autophagy that causes diseases such as depression and schizophrenia?
   a. Cell destruction is not occurring as fast as it is supposed to in neuron cells.
   b. Cell destruction in neurons is accelerated.
   c. Cell destruction occurs abruptly.
   d. Cell destruction stops altogether.

32. Which of the following is MOST likely to occur when autophagy is impaired?
   a. Decrease in mania symptoms
   b. Improvement in Parkinson's disease symptoms
   c. Increase in behaviors associated with personality disorders
   d. Decrease in methamphetamine use

33. A study was performed to see whether new therapies for these seemingly different diseases could be augmented with drugs used for neurodegenerative or neuropsychiatric diseases. Which of the following would be the control group in the study?
   a. The group that did not receive the new therapy.
   b. The group that did receive the therapy.
   c. The drug that had the best results in the study.
   d. The researchers performing the study.

Use the following passage to answer questions 34 through 38.

Class struggle is the key component of Marxist theory. The dominant classes in exploitive societies take possession of surplus labor. Therefore, the subordinate class is critical to production. To maintain surplus and prevent attrition, new workers in such societies often come from generational replacement. This is why women's capacity to have children plays an important role in class society, but also creates a different type of female oppression than occurs in the dominant class. Oppression of women in the dominant classes originates from their role in the maintenance and inheritance of property. In the subordinate classes, the female oppression originates from the women's involvement in the processes that replenish workers, as well as their own work in production.

34. The passage refers to the generational replacement of workers, thus the importance of women being able to bear children. This description refers to which of the following sociological principles?
   a. Intersectionality
   b. Class consciousness
   c. Social reproduction
   d. Intergenerational mobility

35. What is the difference between the status of women in privileged classes and in oppressed classes?
   a. Privileged status is based on inheritance of property; oppressed status is based on reproducing new workers.
   b. Privileged status is based on inheritance of property; oppressed status is based on maintenance of the property of the privileged women.
   c. Privileged women are not oppressed.
   d. The status of both types of women is related to their ability to reproduce new class members.

36. What happens to the infant and maternal mortality rates in oppressed classes?
   a. They are the same as in the privileged class.
   b. They are both higher than in the privileged class.
   c. The infant rate is higher but the maternal rate is the same as in the privileged class.
   d. The maternal rate is higher but the infant rate is the same as in the privileged class.

37. Based on the passage and what you know, which of the following MOST contributes to infant mortality?
   a. Lack of access to health care
   b. The illness experience
   c. Medicalization
   d. The sick role

38. "The dominant classes in exploitive societies take possession of surplus labor. Therefore, the subordinate class is critical to production." Which of the following labels BEST applies to this quote from the passage?

a. Aggression between groups

b. In-group versus out-group

c. Prejudice

d. Discrimination

39. A group of researchers wants to know the effect of a particular treatment on using modeling to change behavior. The results are promising. What is the next step in the research process?

a. Move on to the next problem.

b. Switch the control and experimental groups and repeat the experiment.

c. Double the size of the control group and repeat the experiment.

d. Keep all variables the same and repeat the experiment with a new set of participants.

40. Which of the following identity formation theories BEST describes that a person's self-identity grows out of interpersonal interactions and the perceptions of others?

a. Looking-glass self

b. Role taking

c. Imitation

d. Reference group

41. Which of the following theories focuses on how individuals learn to become criminals but does not concern itself with why they become criminals?

a. Strain theory

b. Differential association

c. Collective behavior

d. Labeling theory

Use the following passage to answer questions 42 through 47.

Recent research has demonstrated that mentally simulating positive intergroup encounters can promote tolerance and more positive intergroup attitudes. A recent study explored the attributional process behind the positive effects. Participants were randomly assigned to three groups. In the first group, participants were instructed to imagine intergroup contact from a first-person perspective. The second group was instructed to imagine the contact from a third-person perspective. Finally, the third group was the control group and received no instructions. Participants from the first-person-perspective group indicated stronger intents to engage in future contact, but the intent was not significantly different from the intent of the control group. Despite this, they did have more positive attitudinal orientation toward out-group encounters after the mental simulation. Participants in the third-person-perspective group also reported stronger intents to engage in future contact, and those intents were significantly stronger than the control group. The findings suggest that attributional processes are important in observing the benefits that are attained from mentally simulating intergroup contact.

42. In this passage, how is attribution theory used?

a. External attribution

b. Interpersonal attribution

c. Common sense attribution

d. Correspondent inference attribution

43. The use of the methodology in the passage in future situations might lead to the reduction of which of the following?

a. Prejudice

b. Self-efficacy

c. Third-person perspective

d. Cognition

44. In this study, the first-person perspective and the third-person perspective were part of which of the following?
   a. Control group
   b. Experimental group
   c. Dependent variables
   d. Independent variables

45. What would be the name of the experimental group in sociological terms?
   a. Primary group
   b. Secondary group
   c. Out-group
   d. Triad

46. Which type of strategy is occurring in this study?
   a. Classical conditioning
   b. Operant conditioning
   c. Observational learning
   d. Reinforcement schedules

47. Which of the following attributional terms would apply if all of the participants in the study had performed the same on both the first-person and third-person treatments?
   a. Consistency
   b. Consensus
   c. Distinctiveness
   d. Expectation

Use the following passage to answer questions 48 through 53.

Many people believe mental illness cannot happen to them. However, one in five adults in America experiences symptoms of a mental health condition each year. Although mental illness affects people in all walks of life, culture plays an important role in its impact. Many minority groups do not receive adequate mental health treatment. This is often due to labeling. Individuals from some racial and ethnic communities who display mental health deficits often experience a more serious disease course than the general population and often receive misdiagnoses.

Another problem for minority groups is the lack of access to quality services. Lack of mental health insurance and inability to pay for prescription medicines (such as antidepressants) often lead to ignored signs of illness. Furthermore, minorities have faced discrimination and biases across social institutions; they often feel that getting help is not worth the additional stress it may bring. Educational support and an increase in quality of service would be valuable in fighting the labeling associated with mental illness in these diverse minority communities.

Mental disorders are extremely common, and the hope is that as more people let go of the shame associated with what they are experiencing, labeling will diminish. The sooner that education, support, and quality services become available for all, the sooner those with a mental illness will find hope.

48. What is another word for *labeling*, as used in this passage?
   a. Stigma
   b. Stereotype
   c. Ethnocentrism
   d. Self-fulfilling prophecy

49. An African-American woman has mild symptoms of bipolar disorder, which she ignores to avoid letting her family and friends know she is sick. Based on the passage, she is attempting to avoid all of the following stages of the illness experience EXCEPT
 a. visiting the appropriate healthcare professionals.
 b. experiencing illness symptoms.
 c. assuming a sick role.
 d. being dependent.

50. The woman in the previous question is MOST likely experiencing which of the following symptoms?
 a. Forgetfulness
 b. Hearing voices
 c. Delusions
 d. Mood swings

51. Broadly, which of the following is BEST demonstrated in this passage?
 a. Social norms
 b. Deindividuation
 c. Social facilitation
 d. Bystander effect

52. Which of the following factors is LEAST likely to change the view of illness in minority social groups?
 a. Biotic factors
 b. Demographic factors
 c. Ideological factors
 d. Environmental factors

53. A group of patients with psychiatric symptoms was divided into four subgroups according to race to see if their existing race-based attitudes about their illness would change if they received a particular treatment. Two of the subgroups were white and two of the subgroups were African American. What is the

MOST likely reason that two subgroups of patients of each race were created instead of just one?
 a. The researchers wanted to increase the number of patients used in the study.
 b. There was a control and an experimental subgroup for each race.
 c. In each subgroup, there was a certain set of symptoms that could be compared.
 d. The second subgroup was added later because the results were not as expected.

Use the following image to answer questions 54 through 56.

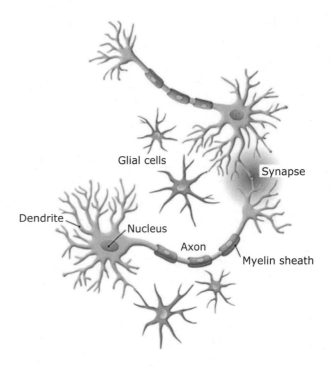

http://www.nichd.nih.gov/news/releases/Pages/012811
-communication-between-brain-cells.aspx.

54. The diagram shows many formations of neurons. How many major parts are there in a typical neuron?
 a. 2
 b. 3
 c. 4
 d. 5

55. Which of the following is another name for the cell body in a nerve cell?

a. Axon

b. Dendrite

c. Processes

d. Soma

56. A man has severe mood swings. Sometimes he is happy, oversexualized, a compulsive shopper, and aggressive. Other times he is sluggish, unhappy, tired, and unmotivated. Which part of the brain's network MOST likely has disruptions that cause these severe mood swings?

a. Neurotransmitters

b. The brain stem

c. Soma

d. The processes

57. A child can hear a sound that an adult cannot hear. Why is this the case?

a. Absolute threshold decreases with age.

b. The adult's auditory pathways are damaged.

c. Feature detection is better in children than in adults.

d. Signal detectors in children function better than in adults.

58. A teacher is using a variable ratio reinforcement schedule as a method to maintain control of her classroom. This is an example of which type of learning?

a. Classical conditioning

b. Operant conditioning

c. Cognitive learning

d. Modeling

59. Which of the following is the term used when a specific recollected experience is incorrectly determined to be the source of a memory?

a. Source monitoring error

b. Neuroplasticity error

c. Trace decay error

d. Interference error

Part 4: Critical Analysis and Reasoning Skills

90 Minutes

53 Questions

Use the following passage to answer questions 1 through 6.

1 The only examples of Joseph Haydn's immense
2 work that the present generation knows are two
3 or three symphonies, rarely and perfunctorily
4 performed. This is the same as saying that we
5 do not know him at all. No musician was ever
6 more prolific or showed a greater wealth of
7 imagination. When we examine this mine of
8 jewels, we are astonished to find at every step a
9 gem which we would have attributed to the
10 invention of some modern or other. We are
11 dazzled by their rays, and where we expect
12 black-and-whites we find pastels grown dim
13 with time.
14   Of Haydn's one hundred and eighteen
15 symphonies, many are simple trifles written
16 from day to day for Prince Esterhazy's little
17 chapel, when the master was musical director
18 there. But after Haydn was called to London by
19 Salomon, a director of concerts, where he had a
20 large orchestra at his disposal, his genius took
21 magnificent flights. Then he wrote great
22 symphonies and in them the clarinets for the
23 first time unfolded the resources from which
24 the modern orchestra has profited so abun-
25 dantly. Originally the clarinet played a humble
26 role, as the name indicates. *Clarinetto* is the
27 diminutive of *clarino*, and the instrument was
28 invented to replace the shrill tones that the
29 trumpet lost as it gained in depth of tone.
30   Like Gluck, Joseph Haydn had the rare
31 advantage of developing constantly. He did not
32 reach the height of his genius until an age when

33   the finest faculties are, ordinarily, in a decline.
34   He astounded the musical world with his
35   *Creation*, in which he displayed a fertility of
36   imagination and a magnificence of orchestral
37   richness that the oratorio had never known
38   before. Emboldened by his success he wrote the
39   *Seasons*, a colossal work, the most varied and
40   the most picturesque in the history of ancient
41   or modern music. In this instance the oratorio
42   is no longer entirely religious. It gives an
43   audacious picture of nature with realistic
44   touches which are astonishing even now. There
45   is an artistic imitation of the different sounds
46   in nature, as the rustling of the leaves, the songs
47   of the birds in the woods and on the farm, and
48   the shrill notes of the insects. Above all that is
49   the translation into music of the profound
50   emotions to which the different aspects of
51   nature give birth, as the freshness of the forests,
52   the stifling heat before a storm, the storm itself,
53   and the wonderful sunset that follows. Then
54   there is a huntsman's chorus which strikes an
55   entirely different note. There are grape harvests,
56   with the mad dances that follow them. There is
57   the winter, with a poignant introduction which
58   reminds us of pages in Schumann. But be
59   reassured, the author does not leave us to the
60   rigors of the cold. He takes us into a farmhouse
61   where the women are spinning and where the
62   peasants are drawn about the fire, listening to a
63   funny tale and laughing immoderately with a
64   gaiety which has never been surpassed.
65   But this gigantic work does not end
66   without giving us a glimpse of Heaven, for with
67   one grand upward burst of flight, Haydn
68   reaches the realms where Handel and
69   Beethoven preceded him. He equals them and
70   ends his picture in a dazzling blaze of light.
    —excerpt from *Musical Memories*
      by Camille Saint-Saëns

1. Which of the following best captures Camille Saint-Saëns' main goal in the passage?
  a. To highlight the innovations of Haydn, unfairly neglected as an important musical master
  b. To argue that Haydn is actually a religious composer
  c. To capture the music of Haydn in vivid pictorial language
  d. To encourage modern musicians to perform Haydn's compositions the way he originally intended

2. Judging from the context, Saint-Saëns' use of the word "picturesque" (line 40) most closely refers to
  a. a realistic, factual story, as opposed to musical compositions based on stories from history, religion, or myth.
  b. an oratorio with the most visually striking backdrop paintings.
  c. an oratorio that creates vivid images in the mind.
  d. a most diverse and unique musical composition.

3. Which of the following passage quotes best supports the argument for the innovative quality of Haydn's work?
  a. "Of Haydn's one hundred and eighteen symphonies, many are simple trifles" (paragraph 2)
  b. "clarinets for the first time unfolded the resources from which the modern orchestra has profited so abundantly" (paragraph 2)
  c. "He did not reach the height of his genius until an age when the finest faculties are, ordinarily, in a decline" (paragraph 3)
  d. "where we expect black-and-whites we find pastels grown dim with time" (paragraph 1)

4. Saint-Saëns cites Haydn's work for Prince Esterhazy, in order to show that

a. wealthy, royal benefactors do not foster great music.

b. creativity requires the right circumstances and atmosphere for genius to really flourish.

c. he can recognize Haydn's flaws and is not merely effusive about his work.

d. creativity is best fostered when a musician does not follow outside influences or trends.

5. Artists of different genres often influence each other. Haydn's *Seasons* was in fact based on a poem of the same title by James Thomson. With which of the following statements about the interplay of the arts would Saint-Saëns most likely agree?

a. The text on which a musical composition is based, whether it's religious, historical, or poetic, is of the utmost importance.

b. Whether it is drama, music, painting, or poetry, the arts are like rival siblings, always seeking to be on the top of a hierarchy of the art forms.

c. One cannot hear a painting, but a piece of music has the power to create a painting in the mind.

d. Music and painting are much more interrelated than music and poetry.

6. In his later years, Haydn suffered a physical decline that made him too weak to play the piano and work out his musical ideas. Suppose Haydn wrote in a letter: "Usually musical ideas are pursuing me, to the point of torture, I cannot escape them, they stand like walls before me. If it's an allegro that pursues me, my pulse keeps beating faster, I can get no sleep. If it's an adagio, then I notice my pulse beating slowly. My imagination plays on me as if I were a clavier." What relevance does this have to the passage?

a. It strengthens the image of Haydn as a prolific musician who showed a great wealth of imagination.

b. It weakens Saint-Saëns' argument that genius is born, not made.

c. It weakens Saint-Saëns' descriptions of Haydn's work as dazzling gems, because Haydn describes his own work as an active thing that lives in a pulse and a heartbeat.

d. It strengthens Saint-Saëns' argument that Haydn suffered from having too many ideas and thus created "simple trifles" alongside masterpieces.

Use the following passage to answer questions 7 through 12.

1 Face to face with an audience, Emma Goldman
2 was a forceful and witty propagandist. Fre-
3 quently she lifted her rapt hearers to heights
4 from which they envisioned a world wholly free
5 and completely delightful. In cold print, how-
6 ever, her lectures reveal little of her dynamic
7 appeal. They are primarily the work of a force-
8 ful agitator: clear, pointed, spirited, but without
9 originality or intellectual rigor.
10   The faithful disciple of Bakunin and
11 Kropotkin, Emma perceived civilization as "a
12 continuous struggle of the individual or of
13 groups of individuals against the State and even
14 against 'society,' that is, against the majority
15 subdued and hypnotized by the State and State
16 worship." This conflict, she argued, was bound
17 to last as long as the state itself, since it was of
18 the very nature of government to be "conserva-
19 tive, static, intolerant of change and opposed to
20 it," while the instinct of the individual was to
21 resent restriction, combat authority, and seek
22 the benefits of innovation.
23   Her definition of anarchism first appeared
24 on the masthead of *Mother Earth* in the issue of
25 April 1910: "The philosophy of a new social

26 order based on liberty unrestrained by man-
27 made law; the theory that all forms of
28 government rest on violence, and are therefore
29 wrong and harmful, as well as unnecessary." In
30 her oft-repeated lecture on the subject she
31 warmly described the benefits to ensue from
32 social revolution: "Anarchism stands for a social
33 order based on the free grouping of individuals
34 for the purpose of producing real social wealth;
35 an order that will guarantee to every human
36 being free access to the earth and full
37 enjoyment of the necessities of life, according
38 to individual desires, tastes, and inclinations."
39   To the end of her life Emma avowed the
40 soundness and practicality of her doctrine. As
41 late as 1934 she declared in *Harper's Magazine*:
42 "I am certain that Anarchism is too vital and
43 too close to human nature ever to die. When
44 the failure of modern dictatorship and authori-
45 tarian philosophies becomes apparent and the
46 realization of failure more general, Anarchism
47 will be vindicated." It was her belief that sooner
48 or later the mass of mankind would perceive
49 the futility of begging for crumbs and would
50 take power into its own hands. Since she
51 scorned political means, she expounded the
52 validity of direct action. This method she
53 defined as the "conscious individual or collec-
54 tive effort to protest against, or remedy, social
55 conditions through the systematic assertion of
56 the economic power of the workers." Once the
57 state and capitalism were destroyed, anarchism
58 would assume the form of free communism,
59 which she described as "a social arrangement
60 based on the principle: To each according to his
61 needs; from each according to his ability." It
62 must be stressed that although the wording is
63 common to all forms of communism, that of
64 Marx and Lenin implies strict centralized
65 authority, while that of Kropotkin and Emma
66 Goldman envisions complete decentralization
67 and the supremacy of the individual.

68   No man who has pondered the concept of
69 the good life will fail to appreciate the ideal
70 propounded by the anarchists. And one who
71 has observed the results of modern dictatorship
72 cannot but sympathize with a vision of the
73 future in which the individual is the prime ben-
74 eficiary of all social activity. Yet life often makes
75 mock of man's noblest dreams. Emma may
76 have been "the daughter of the dream"; her
77 doctrine remains as utopian as it is alluring.
78 There is no gainsaying the fact that modern
79 conditions still favor national and industrial
80 centralization. The philosophy of anarchism
81 appears less tenable today than ever.

—excerpt from *Emma Goldman: Biographical
   Sketch* by Charles Allan Madison

7. Charles Allan Madison's main purpose in this
passage is to
   a. argue that Goldman was a dangerous
   radical.
   b. demonstrate how Goldman failed to create a
   following for her political movement.
   c. discuss Goldman's lifelong pursuit of
   anarchist ideals.
   d. argue that Goldman's lack of intellectual
   rigor led to a failed philosophy.

8. According to the passage, which of the
following is true about Emma Goldman's view
of anarchism?
   a. In the run-up to World War II, fascism
   hindered her faith in humanity to self-
   organize and altered her belief in anarchism.
   b. It is indistinguishable from the communist
   views of Marx and Lenin.
   c. It was considered dangerous to the American
   government and the capitalist system.
   d. It is based on the idea that an individual's
   pursuit and interests often stand in
   contradiction to the pursuits of a
   government.

9. According to the passage, why has the philosophy of anarchism not survived?

   a. Goldman's best work was done through her charismatic speeches, and the only thing that survived her—her unoriginal writing—would not inspire a new generation.

   b. Individuals are inherently violent and are therefore aptly represented by a violent government.

   c. Marxist and Leninist philosophy attracted a greater following.

   d. It is based on utopian ideals that could not stop the reality of national and industrial centralization.

10. According to the information in the passage, which of the following conceptions of Utopia sound closest to the ideal society Goldman advocates?

   a. One in which women rule society

   b. One in which technology improves living and labor conditions so people don't have to "beg for crumbs"

   c. One in which people live in harmony with the natural world

   d. One in which all members only do work they enjoy for the common good

11. Which of the following aspects of transcendentalism aligns with Goldman's conception of anarchy, as outlined in the passage?

      I. The idea that political systems corrupt the individual

      II. The idea that religious belief is based on the inner spirit of the human

      III. The emphasis on individualism

   a. I and II only

   b. III only

   c. I, II, and III

   d. I and III only

12. Which of the following is the best example of Goldman's method of "direct action" (line 52)?

   a. Protesters occupying Wall Street to oppose economic unfairness and corporate greed

   b. Suffragettes marching in order to gain voting rights

   c. Workers lobbying congress to investigate unfair labor practices

   d. An environmentalist chaining herself to a tree

Use the following passage to answer questions 13 through 18.

1   The uproar was appalling, perilous to the
2 eardrums; one feared there was too much
3 sound for the room to hold—that the walls
4 must give way or the ceiling crack. There were
5 high squeals and low squeals, grunts, and wails
6 of agony; there would come a momentary lull,
7 and then a fresh outburst, louder than ever,
8 surging up to a deafening climax. It was too
9 much for some of the visitors—the men would
10 look at each other, laughing nervously, and the
11 women would stand with hands clenched, and
12 the blood rushing to their faces, and the tears
13 starting in their eyes.
14   Meantime, heedless of all these things, the
15 men upon the floor were going about their
16 work. Neither squeals of hogs nor tears of visi-
17 tors made any difference to them; one by one
18 they hooked up the hogs, and one by one with a
19 swift stroke they slit their throats. There was a
20 long line of hogs, with squeals and lifeblood
21 ebbing away together; until at last each started
22 again, and vanished with a splash into a huge
23 vat of boiling water.
24   It was all so very businesslike that one
25 watched it fascinated. It was porkmaking by
26 machinery, porkmaking by applied mathemat-
27 ics. And yet somehow the most matter-of-fact

28 person could not help thinking of the hogs;
29 they were so innocent, they came so very trust-
30 ingly; and they were so very human in their
31 protests—and so perfectly within their rights!
32 They had done nothing to deserve it; and it was
33 adding insult to injury, as the thing was done
34 here, swinging them up in this cold-blooded,
35 impersonal way, without a pretense of apology,
36 without the homage of a tear. Now and then a
37 visitor wept, to be sure; but this slaughtering
38 machine ran on, visitors or no visitors. It was
39 like some horrible crime committed in a dun-
40 geon, all unseen and unheeded, buried out of
41 sight and of memory.
42   One could not stand and watch very long
43 without becoming philosophical, without
44 beginning to deal in symbols and similes, and
45 to hear the hog squeal of the universe. Was it
46 permitted to believe that there was nowhere
47 upon the earth, or above the earth, a heaven for
48 hogs, where they were requited for all this suf-
49 fering? Each one of these hogs was a separate
50 creature. Some were white hogs, some were
51 black; some were brown, some were spotted;
52 some were old, some young; some were long
53 and lean, some were monstrous. And each of
54 them had an individuality of his own, a will of
55 his own, a hope and a heart's desire; each was
56 full of self-confidence, of self-importance, and
57 a sense of dignity. And trusting and strong in
58 faith he had gone about his business, the while
59 a black shadow hung over him and a horrid
60 Fate waited in his pathway. Now suddenly it
61 had swooped upon him, and had seized him by
62 the leg. Relentless, remorseless, it was; all his
63 protests, his screams, were nothing to it—it did
64 its cruel will with him, as if his wishes, his feel-
65 ings, had simply no existence at all; it cut his
66 throat and watched him gasp out his life. And
67 now was one to believe that there was nowhere
68 a god of hogs, to whom this hog personality

69 was precious, to whom these hog squeals and
70 agonies had a meaning? Who would take this
71 hog into his arms and comfort him, reward him
72 for his work well done, and show him the
73 meaning of his sacrifice?
—excerpt from *The Jungle* by Upton Sinclair

13. What is Upton Sinclair's main goal in this passage?
  a. To advocate for vegetarianism
  b. To argue that the industrialization of food systems is inherently wrong
  c. To expose the inhumane practices of the pork industry
  d. To show how the fear of death can swoop upon an individual at any moment

14. According to Sinclair, why must one deal with symbols and similes?
  a. Dealing with the facts of the situation is too disturbing.
  b. It captures the situation of the slaughterhouse more vividly than mere description.
  c. It is difficult to face industrial slaughter; one wants to give it meaning.
  d. The rhythmic nature of the slaughter machine is mesmerizing and makes the mind wander.

15. Sinclair mentions the "god of hogs" (line 68) in order to
  a. say something comical and lighten the mood of his philosophizing.
  b. highlight the issue of the morality of eating an animal.
  c. appeal to a higher power to stop the slaughter of hogs.
  d. express the wish that the hog be treated with care in its life and dignity in its death.

16. Which of the following is the best argument AGAINST Sinclair's sentiments in the concluding paragraph?
   a. Industrial farms are a vital component in creating enough food to sustain the human population.
   b. Hogs squeal for a number of reasons, including when they enjoy rolling in the mud.
   c. We project human emotion onto animals, which is why we have pets, but a hog does not possess something like hope or a sense of self-importance.
   d. These pigs were raised for slaughter; they would not exist if the machine did not exist.

17. If the following sentence were added to the final paragraph, what effect would it have on the passage? "As if in answer to the question, looking down this room, one saw a line of dangling hogs a hundred yards in length; and for every yard, there was a man whose arms were working as if a demon were after him."
   a. It would strengthen the idea of a "hog heaven" to also introduce the idea of a "hog hell."
   b. It would weaken the passage because it brings the discussion out of the philosophical hog heaven and back to the reality of the industrial farm.
   c. It would strengthen the passage because it brings the discussion out of the philosophical hog heaven and back to the reality of the industrial farm.
   d. It would weaken the passage because it doesn't provide a direct answer to the final question of the passage.

18. Which of the following critical statements that deal with the political and ethical aspects of eating and the industrial farm speak most directly to the issues discussed in the passage?
   a. "We are surrounded by an enterprise of degradation, cruelty, and killing which rivals anything that the Third Reich was capable of, indeed dwarfs it, in that ours is an enterprise without end, self-regenerating, bringing rabbits, rats, poultry, livestock ceaselessly into the world for the purpose of killing them." (J. M. Coetzee)
   b. "The way we eat represents our most profound engagement with the natural world." (Michael Pollan)
   c. "If possessing a higher degree of intelligence does not entitle one human to use another for his or her own ends, how can it entitle humans to exploit non-humans for the same purpose?" (Peter Singer)
   d. "Our sustenance now comes from misery. We know that if someone offers to show us a film on how our meat is produced, it will be a horror film." (Jonathan Safran Foer)

Use the following passage to answer questions 19 through 24.

1 It must be remembered that Spain, in the years
2 following her brilliant conquests of the fif-
3 teenth and sixteenth centuries, lost strength
4 and vigor through the corruption at home
5 induced by the unearned wealth that flowed
6 into the mother country from the colonies, and
7 by the draining away of her best blood. Nor did
8 her sons ever develop that economic spirit
9 which is the permanent foundation of all
10 empire, but they let the wealth of the Indies
11 flow through their country, principally to
12 London and Amsterdam, there to form in more
13 practical hands the basis of the British and
14 Dutch colonial empires.

15   The priest and the soldier were supreme,
16 so her best sons took up either the cross or the
17 sword to maintain her dominion in the distant
18 colonies, a movement which, long continued,
19 spelled for her a form of national suicide. The
20 soldier expended his strength and generally laid
21 down his life on alien soil, leaving no fit succes-
22 sor of his own stock to carry on the work
23 according to his standards. The priest under the
24 celibate system, in its better days left no off-
25 spring at all and in the days of its corruption
26 none bred and reared under the influences that
27 make for social and political progress. The dark
28 chambers of the Inquisition stifled all advance
29 in thought, so the civilization and the culture of
30 Spain, as well as her political system, settled
31 into rigid forms to await only the inevitable
32 process of stagnation and decay. In her proud-
33 est hour an old soldier, who had lost one of his
34 hands fighting her battles against the Turk at
35 Lepanto, employed the other in writing the
36 masterpiece of her literature, which is really a
37 caricature of the nation.
38   There is much in the career of Spain that
39 calls to mind the dazzling beauty of her "dark-
40 glancing daughters," with its early bloom, its
41 startling—almost morbid—brilliance, and its
42 premature decay. Rapid and brilliant was her
43 rise, gradual and inglorious her steady decline,
44 from the bright morning when the banners of
45 Castile and Aragon were flung triumphantly
46 from the battlements of the Alhambra, to the
47 short summer, not so long gone, when at Cavite
48 and Santiago with swift, decisive havoc the last
49 ragged remnants of the once world-dominating
50 power were blown into space and time, to hover
51 disembodied there, a lesson and a warning to
52 future generations. Whatever her final place in
53 the records of mankind, whether as the pioneer
54 of modern civilization or the buccaneer of the
55 nations or, as would seem most likely, a goodly

56 mixture of both, she has at least—with the
57 exception only of her great mother, Rome—
58 furnished the most instructive lessons in politi-
59 cal pathology yet recorded, and the advice to
60 students of world progress to familiarize them-
61 selves with her history is even more apt today
62 than when it first issued from the encyclopedic
63 mind of Macaulay nearly a century ago. Hardly
64 had she reached the zenith of her power when
65 the disintegration began, and one by one her
66 brilliant conquests dropped away, to leave her
67 alone in her faded splendor, with naught but
68 her vaunting pride left, another "Niobe of
69 nations." In the countries more in contact with
70 the trend of civilization and more susceptible to
71 revolutionary influences from the mother
72 country this separation came from within,
73 while in the remoter parts the archaic and out
74 grown system dragged along until a stronger
75 force from without destroyed it.

—excerpt from *Noli Me Tangere* by José Rizal

19. The best title for this passage would be
   a. "Spain and Its Conquests."
   b. "The Priest and the Soldier."
   c. "Progress and the Spanish Inquisition."
   d. "The Fall of the Spanish Empire."

20. Judging from the context, "political pathology"
   (lines 58–59) could best be described as
   a. the expansion of the mother country into
      many colonies.
   b. the systemic problems that lead to the
      decline of a nation.
   c. the lies that the ruling class tell themselves
      and the nation's citizens.
   d. the plague that decimated Spain's
      population while also destroying its political
      structure.

21. Rizal refers to the "celibacy of priests" as a problem for the Spanish Empire. What does he most likely mean?

   a. Spanish society was overrun with celibate priests, to the extent that it could not produce enough offspring and sustain a population in its new colonies, so the empire waned.

   b. Priests could not produce more priests, so when the empire expanded, the colonies were left without an important part of the motherland's culture.

   c. The "celibacy of priests" is a metaphor for the stifling nature of the religion that held back political and cultural progress in the Spanish empire.

   d. The priesthood produced a system of corruption that matched that of the empire's political leaders.

22. When Rizal refers to the old soldier who wrote the masterpiece of Spain's literature, he refers to Cervantes' *Don Quixote*. The historical fact that one of the masterpieces of Spain came out of this time period does not align with his argument that the Inquisition stifled cultural progress. Which of the following phrases helps mitigate this inconvenient historical fact?

   I. Framing it as Spain's "proudest hour"

   II. Emphasizing that the soldier lost one hand

   III. Emphasizing that it was a caricature

   a. I, II, and III

   b. I only

   c. II and III

   d. III only

23. The Greek myth of Niobe portrays a mother who brags about her plentiful children to the Titan Leto, who only has two children, Apollo and Artemis. Apollo then kills all of Niobe's sons, and Artemis kills all of Niobe's daughters.

Niobe becomes a symbol of mourning. According to the reference in the passage, what relevance does this myth have to Spain's decline?

   a. The mother country was too boastful of its colonies.

   b. Spain had too many colonies to adequately care for.

   c. Spain became mournful for the loss of its greatness as an empire.

   d. Spain's colonies were destroyed from within by "national suicide."

24. Which of the following factors that led to the fall of the Roman Empire also led to the fall of the Spanish Empire, as outlined in the passage?

   a. Invasions by barbarian tribes

   b. Reliance on slave labor

   c. The rise of a competing empire

   d. Government corruption

Use the following passage to answer questions 25 through 30.

1   Except it be a lover, no one is more interesting
2   as an object of study than a student. Shakespeare
3   might have made him a fourth in his immortal
4   group. The lunatic with his fixed idea, the poet
5   with his fine frenzy, the lover with his frantic
6   idolatry, and the student aflame with the desire
7   for knowledge are of "imagination all compact."
8   To an absorbing passion, a whole-souled devo-
9   tion, must be joined an enduring energy, if the
10   student is to become a devotee of the gray-eyed
11   goddess to whose law his services are bound.
12   Like the quest of the Holy Grail, the quest of
13   Minerva is not for all. For the one, the pure life;
14   for the other, what Milton calls "a strong pro-
15   pensity of nature." Here again the student often
16   resembles the poet—he is born, not made.
17   While the resultant of two molding forces, the
18   accidental, external conditions, and the hidden

19   germinal energies, which produce in each one
20   of us national, family, and individual traits, the
21   true student possesses in some measure a
22   divine spark which sets at naught their laws.
23   Like the Snark, he defies definition, but there
24   are three unmistakable signs by which you may
25   recognize the genuine article from a Boojum—
26   an absorbing desire to know the truth, an
27   unswerving steadfastness in its pursuit, and an
28   open, honest heart, free from suspicion, guile,
29   and jealousy.
30   At the outset do not be worried about this
31   big question—Truth. It is a very simple matter
32   if each one of you starts with the desire to get as
33   much as possible. No human being is
34   constituted to know the truth, the whole truth,
35   and nothing but the truth; and even the best of
36   men must be content with fragments, with
37   partial glimpses, never the full fruition. In this
38   unsatisfied quest the attitude of mind, the
39   desire, the thirst—a thirst that from the soul
40   must rise!—the fervent longing, are the be-all
41   and the end-all. What is the student but a lover
42   courting a fickle mistress who ever eludes his
43   grasp? In this very elusiveness is brought out his
44   second great characteristic—steadfastness of
45   purpose. Unless from the start the limitations
46   incident to our frail human faculties are frankly
47   accepted, nothing but disappointment awaits
48   you. The truth is the best you can get with your
49   best endeavor, the best that the best men
50   accept—with this you must learn to be satisfied,
51   retaining at the same time with due humility an
52   earnest desire for an ever larger portion. Only
53   by keeping the mind plastic and receptive does
54   the student escape perdition. It is not, as
55   Charles Lamb remarks, that some people do
56   not know what to do with truth when it is
57   offered to them, but the tragic fate is to reach,
58   after years of patient search, a condition of
59   mind-blindness in which the truth is not recog-
60   nized, though it stares you in the face. This can

61   never happen to a man who has followed step
62   by step the growth of a truth, and who knows
63   the painful phases of its evolution. It is one of
64   the great tragedies of life that every truth has to
65   struggle to acceptance against honest but mind-
66   blind students. Harvey knew his
67   contemporaries well, and for twelve successive
68   years demonstrated the circulation of the blood
69   before daring to publish the facts on which the
70   truth was based.
71   Only steadfastness of purpose and humil-
72   ity enable the student to shift his position to
73   meet the new conditions in which new truths
74   are born, or old ones modified beyond recogni-
75   tion. And, thirdly, the honest heart will keep
76   him in touch with his fellow students, and fur-
77   nish that sense of comradeship without which
78   he travels an arid waste alone.
     —excerpt from *The Student Life*
        by William Osler

25. According to the passage, which of the
       following are important qualities that the
       student must possess?
       a. Ingenuity and a suspicion of accepted truths
       b. Ambition and a thirst for the pure life
       c. Persistence and a captivating desire for
            knowledge
       d. Courage and an intense love of the
            unexpected

26. Osler mentions Shakespeare's "immortal
       group" (line 3). What is the relationship
       between the lunatic and the student, according
       to him?
       a. Both deal with the imaginary.
       b. The lunatic's ideas are static, whereas the
            student's are ever changing.
       c. One deals with ideas, whereas the other deals
            with knowledge.
       d. Both have a fervent focus.

27. Osler cites the work of physician Harvey in order to show that

a. one must make absolutely sure of the facts before publishing.

b. someone may know a truth but may not have the courage to share it.

c. a new truth that changes how we see the world will be met with opposition.

d. facts will always lead to the truth, even if it takes time.

28. Osler discusses the "Snark" as the "true student" and the "Boojum" as the imposter. It is a reference to Lewis Carroll's nonsense poem, "The Hunting of the Snark," in which a crew sets sail to find the fictional creature. In the end, the crew catch what they think is a Snark but which turns out to be a Boojum, a dangerous creature that causes its hunter to fade away. How else might this tale relate to the student and his journey?

a. It emphasizes the idea of the student's journey as the unsatisfied quest for truth.

b. It suggests that the student may be haunted by his imagination when searching for truth.

c. It emphasizes that a student should not lose himself in the pursuit of knowledge.

d. It shows that the hunt for knowledge can at times be nonsensical.

29. According to the passage, which of the following quotes about truth might Osler agree is the most relevant to the student?

a. Schopenhauer's "All truth passes through three stages. First, it is ridiculed. Second, it is violently opposed. Third, it is accepted as being self-evident."

b. Whitman's "Whatever satisfies the soul is truth."

c. Angelou's "There's a world of difference between truth and facts. Facts can obscure the truth."

d. Descartes's "If you would be a real seeker after truth, it is necessary that at least once in your life you doubt, as far as possible, all things."

30. Aristotle said, "The roots of education are bitter but the fruit is sweet." If we understand the "fruit" to be the truth gained through the learning process, which of the following would most likely be Osler's response?

a. One must have a fervid love for the cultivation of roots and a thirst for the fruit.

b. Some people will not know what to do with the fruit when it is offered them.

c. To the true student, the roots of education are sweet and the fruit is bitter.

d. The true student may skip the cultivation process and go directly to the fruit.

Use the following passage to answer questions 31 through 36.

1   There is no question that the facts of crowd
2   excitement, of class, caste, race, and national
3   consciousness, show the way in which the indi-
4   vidual members of a group are, or seem to be,
5   dominated, at certain moments and under cer-
6   tain circumstances, by the group as a whole.
7   Worms gives to this fact, and the phenomena
8   that accompany it, the title "collective con-
9   sciousness." This gives the problem a name, to
10 be sure, but not a solution. What the purpose of
11 sociology requires is a description and an
12 explanation. Under what conditions, precisely,
13 does this phenomenon of collective conscious-
14 ness arise? What are the mechanisms—physical,
15 physiological, and social—by which the group
16 imposes its control, or what seems to be con-
17 trol, upon the individual members of the
18 group?
19   This question had arisen and been answered
20 by political philosophers, in terms of political

21 philosophy, long before sociology attempted to
22 give an objective account of the matter. Two
23 classic phrases, Aristotle's "Man is a political
24 animal" and Hobbes's "War of each against all,"
25 *omnes bellum omnium*, measure the range and
26 divergence of the schools upon this topic.
27   According to Hobbes, the existing moral
28 and political order—that is to say the organiza-
29 tion of control—is in any community a mere
30 artifact, a control resting on consent, supported
31 by a prudent calculation of consequences, and
32 enforced by an external power. Aristotle, on the
33 other hand, taught that man was made for life
34 in society just as the bee is made for life in the
35 hive. The relations between the sexes, as well as
36 those between mother and child, are manifestly
37 predetermined in the physiological organiza-
38 tion of the individual man and woman.
39 Furthermore, man is, by his instincts and his
40 inherited dispositions, predestined to a social
41 existence beyond the intimate family circle.
42 Society must be conceived, therefore, as a part
43 of nature, like a beaver's dam or the nests of
44 birds.
45   As a matter of fact, man and society pres-
46 ent themselves in a double aspect. They are at
47 the same time products of nature and of
48 human artifice. Just as a stone hammer in the
49 hand of a savage may be regarded as an artifi-
50 cial extension of the natural man, so tools,
51 machinery, technical and administrative
52 devices, including the formal organization of
53 government and the informal "political
54 machine," may be regarded as more or less arti-
55 ficial extensions of the natural social group.
56   So far as this is true, the conflict between
57 Hobbes and Aristotle is not absolute. Society is
58 a product both of nature and of design, of
59 instinct and of reason. If, in its formal aspect,
60 society is therefore an artifact, it is one which
61 connects up with and has its roots in nature
62 and in human nature.

63   This does not explain social control but
64 simplifies the problem of corporate action. It
65 makes clear, at any rate, that as members of
66 society, men act as they do elsewhere from
67 motives they do not fully comprehend, in order
68 to fulfill aims of which they are but dimly or
69 not at all conscious. Men are activated, in short,
70 not merely by interests, in which they are con-
71 scious of the end they seek, but also by instincts
72 and sentiments, the source and meaning of
73 which they do not clearly comprehend.
—excerpt from *Introduction to the Science of Sociology* by Park and Burgess

31. Park and Burgess's use of the phrase "corporate action" (line 64) most closely means
   a. the actions undertaken by business executives.
   b. the movements of the human body that are at times involuntary.
   c. social control in its simplest form.
   d. the actions of a group.

32. What is the irony in Park and Burgess's conclusions in the final paragraph about "collective consciousness"?
   a. The condition of "collective consciousness" can arise through people's unconscious decisions.
   b. A series of individual wills could be exactly the same as the collective will of an entire group.
   c. The collective consciousness is actually a thing that gets scattered.
   d. People use the idea as a means of social control, but it is what leads to riots.

33. What is the logical relationship Park and Burgess present between the "stone hammer" and the "political machine" (lines 48–54)?

a. The political machine represents modern-day society, which evolved from primitive man, represented by the stone hammer.

b. They are both extensions of the human being—one is an extension of the individual, the other of the group.

c. They are opposites—the stone hammer represents the simple, while the "political machine" represents the complex.

d. The stone hammer was a primitive weapon, and the "political machine" is a modern weapon.

34. Which of the following statements best expresses Aristotle's idea of society as outlined in the passage?

a. Humans are predestined to interact with society.

b. Human society works cooperatively, like the interworking parts of a machine.

c. Mothers and children form the basis of human society.

d. Human society is like a beaver's dam that stops the flow of the natural order of things.

35. Psychologist Carl Jung coined the term "collective unconscious," which describes the part of the unconscious made up of inherited ancestral memory and concepts that are universal to all humans. What relevance does this information have to the idea of the collective consciousness as outlined in the passage?

a. It strengthens the idea of a group motivated by similar unconscious desires or instincts.

b. It weakens the idea that consciousness is required to motivate a group.

c. It weakens the idea that people are dominated by a group because they are dominated by their ancestors instead.

d. It strengthens the idea that individuals cannot be influenced by outside forces unless they offer their consent.

36. Which of the following would NOT be an example of collective consciousness, as outlined in the passage?

a. The shared beliefs of a religious sect

b. The harmony of a symphony

c. The inclination to cheer at a political rally

d. Being quiet in a library so as not to disturb others

Use the following passage to answer questions 37 through 41.

1   Between me and the other world there is ever
2   an unasked question: unasked by some through
3   feelings of delicacy; by others through the diffi-
4   culty of rightly framing it. All, nevertheless,
5   flutter round it. They approach me in a half-
6   hesitant sort of way, eye me curiously or com-
7   passionately, and then, instead of saying
8   directly, *How does it feel to be a problem?* they
9   say, *I know an excellent colored man in my town;*
10   or, *I fought at Mechanicsville;* or, *Do not these*
11   *Southern outrages make your blood boil?* At these
12   I smile, or am interested, or reduce the boiling
13   to a simmer, as the occasion may require. To the
14   real question, *How does it feel to be a problem?* I
15   answer seldom a word.
16   And yet, being a problem is a strange
17   experience,—peculiar even for one who has
18   never been anything else, save perhaps in baby-
19   hood and in Europe. It is in the early days of
20   rollicking boyhood that the revelation first
21   bursts upon one, all in a day, as it were. I

22 remember well when the shadow swept across
23 me. I was a little thing, away up in the hills of
24 New England, where the dark Housatonic
25 winds between Hoosac and Taghkanic to the
26 sea. In a wee wooden schoolhouse, something
27 put it into the boys' and girls' heads to buy gor-
28 geous visiting-cards—ten cents a package—and
29 exchange. The exchange was merry, till one girl,
30 a tall newcomer, refused my card,—refused it
31 peremptorily, with a glance. Then it dawned
32 upon me with a certain suddenness that I was
33 different from the others; or like, mayhap, in
34 heart and life and longing, but shut out from
35 their world by a vast veil. I had thereafter no
36 desire to tear down that veil, to creep through; I
37 held all beyond it in common contempt, and
38 lived above it in a region of blue sky and great
39 wandering shadows. That sky was bluest when I
40 could beat my mates at examination-time, or
41 beat them at a foot-race, or even beat their
42 stringy heads. Alas, with the years all this fine
43 contempt began to fade; for the words I longed
44 for, and all their dazzling opportunities, were
45 theirs, not mine. But they should not keep these
46 prizes, I said; some, all, I would wrest from
47 them. Just how I would do it I could never
48 decide: by reading law, by healing the sick, by
49 telling the wonderful tales that swam in my
50 head,—some way. With other black boys the
51 strife was not so fiercely sunny: their youth
52 shrunk into tasteless sycophancy, or into silent
53 hatred of the pale world about them and mock-
54 ing distrust of everything white; or wasted itself
55 in a bitter cry, Why did God make me an out-
56 cast and a stranger in mine own house? The
57 shades of the prison-house closed round about
58 us all: walls strait and stubborn to the whitest,
59 but relentlessly narrow, tall, and unscalable to
60 sons of night who must plod darkly on in resig-

61 nation, or beat unavailing palms against the
62 stone, or steadily, half hopelessly, watch the
63 streak of blue above.

—excerpt from *The Souls of Black Folk* by
W. E. B. Du Bois

37. Judging from the context, the "vast veil" (line 35) could best be described as
  a. a disguise that made the exterior world elusive.
  b. an invisible barrier that separated blacks from whites.
  c. a thin, gauzy material used for segregation in classrooms.
  d. a mask that the author lived behind.

38. What does Du Bois mean by living in the "blue sky and great wandering shadows" (lines 38–39)?
  a. One must rise above racism.
  b. He became absentminded in order to forget the "problem."
  c. One must always look up and see the bright side of things.
  d. He lived mostly in his imagination.

39. Du Bois's discussion of the "prison-house" most likely argues that
  a. there is a racial bias in the criminal justice system.
  b. racial inequality is a prison for both whites and blacks in America.
  c. language is racially tinged by images of light and dark.
  d. the barrier between races is insurmountable.

40. Which quote from W. E. B. Du Bois most closely matches the sentiment of the passage?

    a. "To be a poor man is hard, but to be a poor race in a land of dollars is the very bottom of hardships."

    b. "The chief problem in any community cursed with crime is not the punishment of the criminals, but the preventing of the young from being trained to crime."

    c. "It is a peculiar sensation, this double-consciousness, this sense of always looking at one's self through the eyes of others, of measuring one's soul by the tape of a world that looks on in amused contempt and pity."

    d. "The problem of the twentieth century is the problem of the color-line,—the relation of the darker to the lighter races of men."

41. Prominent black Civil Rights leader Booker T. Washington once said of race relations in America, "In all things purely social we can be as separate as the five fingers, and yet one as the hand in all things essential to mutual progress." Based on the passage, which of the following would be Du Bois's LEAST likely response?

    a. One cannot separate blacks and whites "in all things social" because we are members of the same society with the same concerns.

    b. The only definition of progress should be to tear down the barrier between blacks and whites.

    c. That which separates us also imprisons us; progress cannot be made from the prison house.

    d. When one finger is weighed down by the dazzling rings of opportunity, the course of progress shifts in that direction.

Use the following passage to answer questions 42 through 47.

1   A town, such as London, where a man may
2   wander for hours together without reaching the
3   beginning of the end, without meeting the
4   slightest hint which could lead to the inference
5   that there is open country within reach, is a
6   strange thing. This colossal centralization, this
7   heaping together of two and a half millions of
8   human beings at one point, has multiplied the
9   power of this two and a half millions a hun-
10   dredfold; has raised London to the commercial
11   capital of the world, created the giant docks and
12   assembled the thousand vessels that continually
13   cover the Thames. I know nothing more impos-
14   ing than the view which the Thames offers
15   during the ascent from the sea to London
16   Bridge. The masses of buildings, the wharves
17   on both sides, especially from Woolwich
18   upwards, the countless ships along both shores,
19   crowding ever closer and closer together, until,
20   at last, only a narrow passage remains in the
21   middle of the river, a passage through which
22   hundreds of steamers shoot by one another; all
23   this is so vast, so impressive, that a man cannot
24   collect himself, but is lost in the marvel of
25   England's greatness before he sets foot upon
26   English soil.
27   But the sacrifices which all this has cost
28   become apparent later. After roaming the
29   streets of the capital a day or two, making head-
30   way with difficulty through the human turmoil
31   and the endless lines of vehicles, after visiting
32   the slums of the metropolis, one realizes for the
33   first time that these Londoners have been
34   forced to sacrifice the best qualities of their
35   human nature, to bring to pass all the marvels
36   of civilization which crowd their city; that a
37   hundred powers which slumbered within them

38 have remained inactive, have been suppressed
39 in order that a few might be developed more
40 fully and multiply through union with those of
41 others. The very turmoil of the streets has
42 something repulsive, something against which
43 human nature rebels. The hundreds of thou-
44 sands of all classes and ranks crowding past
45 each other, are they not all human beings with
46 the same qualities and powers, and with the
47 same interest in being happy? And have they
48 not, in the end, to seek happiness in the same
49 way, by the same means? And still they crowd
50 by one another as though they had nothing in
51 common, nothing to do with one another, and
52 their only agreement is the tacit one, that each
53 keep to his own side of the pavement, so as not
54 to delay the opposing streams of the crowd,
55 while it occurs to no man to honor another
56 with so much as a glance. The brutal indiffer-
57 ence, the unfeeling isolation of each in his
58 private interest becomes the more repellant and
59 offensive, the more these individuals are
60 crowded together, within a limited space. And,
61 however much one may be aware that this
62 isolation of the individual, this narrow self-
63 seeking is the fundamental principle of our
64 society everywhere, it is nowhere so shamelessly
65 barefaced, so self-conscious as just here in the
66 crowding of the great city. The dissolution of
67 mankind into monads, of which each one has a
68 separate principle, the world of atoms, is here
69 carried out to its utmost extreme.
70 　　　Hence it comes, too, that the social war,
71 the war of each against all, is here openly
72 declared. Just as in Stirner's recent book, people
73 regard each other only as useful objects; each
74 exploits the other, and the end of it all is, that
75 the stronger treads the weaker under foot.
　　　—excerpt from *The Condition of the Working-*
　　　　Class in England in 1844 by Frederick Engels

42. The passage's central thesis is that
　　a. science has reduced the human being to a collection of atoms.
　　b. a large group of people, like those found in a city, will necessarily suffer from groupthink.
　　c. the industrial-urban model of human existence sacrifices something essentially human for the individual.
　　d. it is ironic that people choose to stay squeezed into a city when the "open country" is only just miles away.

43. Judging from the context, the "human turmoil" (line 30) could best be described as
　　a. the anguish one feels when surrounded by the cityscape.
　　b. the noise and commotion of the people of the city.
　　c. the cost of what is lost of one's humanity in a city.
　　d. the war of each individual against the other.

44. Which of the following aspects of city life would Engels agree is a good thing?
　　a. The camaraderie felt among its citizens
　　b. The intellectual life of the city
　　c. The hustle and bustle of city streets
　　d. None of the above

45. According to Engels, "narrow self-seeking" is a fundamental principle of our society because
　　a. city life creates a brutal indifference within people.
　　b. people are creatures of evolution, each seeking to gain favor in the survival of the fittest.
　　c. people have had to sacrifice their best qualities of human nature in order to create the marvels of civilization.
　　d. isolation is the most natural human quality.

46. Which of the following sights might have changed his conclusions about society if Engels had seen it in his walk about London?
a. The grave of Charles Dickens
b. An architectural tour
c. A British library
d. A homeless shelter

47. Which of the following examples of animal behavior most closely matches Engel's characterization of humans in the city he describes?
a. The rhesus monkey that fights members of its troop for dominance in its social hierarchy
b. The bees that engage in cooperative work to build honeycombs
d. The vampire bat that engages in "reciprocal altruism" by sharing food with starving members of its species
d. The bonobo that aids an injured member of its species

Use the following passage to answer questions 48 through 53.

1   In Philadelphia the new movement has some
2   powerful allies, among whom should be promi-
3   nently mentioned Thomas Eakins, a pupil of
4   Gérôme, and at present professor in the Phila-
5   delphia Academy of Art. One of Mr. Eakins's
6   most ambitions paintings represents a surgical
7   operation before a class in anatomy. It is char-
8   acterized by so many excellent artistic qualities,
9   that one regrets that the work as a whole fails to
10 satisfy. Admirable draughtsman as this painter
11 is, one is surprised that in the arrangement of
12 the figures the perspective should have been so
13 ineffective that the mother is altogether too
14 small for the rest of the group, and the figure of
15 the patient so indistinct that it is difficult to tell

16 exactly the part of the body upon which the
17 surgeon is performing the operation. The
18 monochromatic tone of the composition is,
19 perhaps, intentional, in order to concentrate
20 the effect on the bloody thigh and the crimson
21 finger of the operating professor. But as it is, the
22 attention is at once and so entirely directed on
23 that reeking hand as to convey the impression
24 that such concentration was the sole purpose of
25 the painting. In similar paintings by Ribeira,
26 Regnault, and other artists of the horrible, as
27 vivid a result is obtained without sacrificing the
28 light and color in the other parts of the picture;
29 and the effect, while no less intense, is, there-
30 fore, less staring and loud. As to the propriety
31 of introducing into our art a class of subjects
32 hitherto confined to a few of the more brutal
33 artists of the Old World, the question may well
34 be left to the decision of the public. In color Mr.
35 Eakins effects a low tone that is sometimes
36 almost monochromatic, but has very few equals
37 in the country in drawing of the figure. Some
38 of his portraits are strongly characteristic, and
39 give remarkable promise. Miss Emily Sartain is
40 devoting herself with good success to *genre* and
41 portraiture; and Miss Mary Cassatt merits more
42 extended notice and earnest praise for the glory
43 of color and the superb treatment and compo-
44 sition of some of her works.
45   When we review the various forces now
46 actively at work to hasten forward the progress
47 of American art, we see that they are, with one
48 or two exceptions, still immature; while, on the
49 other hand, the sum of their influence is such
50 as to prove that they are already sufficiently well
51 established to give abundant promise of vitality,
52 and of a career of success that seems destined to
53 carry the arts to a degree of excellence never
54 before seen in America. While the ideal is a
55 more prominent feature of our art than for-
56 merly, the tide also sets strongly toward realism,
57 together with a clearer practical knowledge of

58 technique. And while we do not discover
59 marked original power in the artists who repre-
60 sent the new movement, we find in them a self-
61 reliance and a sturdiness of purpose which
62 renders them potential in establishing the end
63 they have in view. It is to their successors that
64 we must look for the founding of a school that
65 shall be at once native in origin, and powerful
66 in the employment of the material to express
67 the ideal.

—excerpt from *Art in America* by Samuel
Greene Wheeler (S. G. W.) Benjamin

48. The main purpose of the passage is
   a. to characterize a new movement in
      American art.
   b. to emphasize the importance of color in
      realistic paintings.
   c. to admonish Eakins's use of brutal subject
      matter.
   d. to argue that subject is as important as
      technique in painting.

49. What does Benjamin's use of the word
   "propriety" (line 30) most likely refer to?
   a. He is suggesting that art is meant to be
      beautiful.
   b. He suggests that a surgical theater may be an
      objectionable subject for an American
      audience.
   c. He is emphasizing the idea that art is meant
      to be instructive.
   d. He is questioning whether it is right to
      introduce new subject matter into a
      movement that is still in its infancy.

50. Which of the following criticisms of Benjamin's
   argument is the WEAKEST?
   a. The discussion of this "new movement"
      spends too much time criticizing one
      painting, which Benjamin does not even
      provide the name for.
   b. The discussion of the female painters seems
      tacked on to the end of the first paragraph,
      as if to pay lip service to the existence of
      women while not actually discussing their
      work.
   c. Benjamin is overly concerned with American
      art, while neglecting the art of other
      cultures.
   d. Realism and idealism are in conflict, yet
      Benjamin seems to say that the "new
      movement" embodies both—the
      summations of the final paragraph are
      contradictory and unclear.

51. Benjamin does not provide a name for the
   "new movement." Based on the descriptions in
   the passage, which of the following paintings
   might be included in this "new movement"?
   a. A painting that draws attention to social
      issues of the working class and the poor
   b. A painting that seeks to capture moods in
      color and abstract form
   c. A painting that seeks to represent its subjects
      realistically without artificial embellishments
   d. A painting that seeks to capture visible
      brushstrokes and the changing qualities of
      light

52. More than a decade later, Eakins painted a similar composition of a surgical operation called *The Agnew Clinic*, with much brighter lighting and surgeons all dressed in white overcoats. It reflected the new practices of antiseptic surgery established in the intervening years between the two paintings. How does this information affect Benjamin's discussion of the earlier Eakins painting?

    a. It weakens the idea that Eakins was an "admirable draughtsman," because he painted the same composition again.

    b. It strengthens Benjamin's analysis that Eakins sacrificed color in most of the painting in order to highlight the blood.

    c. It weakens Benjamin's criticism that Eakins sacrificed light, because he may have captured the realism of an operation that was not very well lit.

    d. It strengthens Benjamin's argument, because Eakins did, in fact, change his style, adding more light to his paintings.

53. Which of the following aesthetic theories seem most important for the author's view of art?

    a. Mimetic—that art is representation, a mirror held up to the world

    b. Pragmatic—that art should teach people something

    c. Expressive—that art is an expression of the artist, a mirror held up to "the self"

    d. Objective—that art should be about art itself, about paint and the artist's brushstrokes

Answers

Part 1: Biological and Biochemical Foundations of Living Systems

  1. b. As stated in the passage, the addition of multiple ubiquitin groups to p53 (and to proteins in general) directs it to the 26S proteasome complex and results in its clearance from the cell.

  2. a. As stated in the passage, protein phosphorylation often occurs in the cytosol, which is the aqueous phase of the cell.

  3. c. As stated in the passage, covalent modifications are dynamic, whereas proteolytic cleavage is irreversible.

  4. d. Restriction enzyme digest is a method to process DNA for cloning or analysis.

  5. b. Protein phosphorylation typically occurs on serine, threonine, and tyrosine residues.

  6. a. As stated in the passage, glucokinase catalyzes the phosphorylation of glucose to glucose 6-phosphate, which is the first step of glycolysis, or the breakdown of glucose.

  7. d. This is the correct choice. As stated in the passage, hexokinase I and glucokinase (hexokinase IV) catalyze the same reaction (phosphorylation of glucose to glucose 6-phosphate) in different cells of the body. They are two of four hexokinase isozymes (along with hexokinase II and III). *Isozyme* is the term for two different enzymes that catalyze the same reaction.

  8. b. As stated in the passage, glucokinase converts glucose to glycogen in the liver, and this process is called glycogenesis.

  9. c. This is the correct choice. Allosteric enzymes function through reversible, noncovalent binding of regulatory compounds called allosteric effectors.

10. b. This is the correct choice. Hexokinase I reaches half of its maximum reaction rate when the concentration of glucose is well below 5 mM, whereas the maximum reaction of glucokinase is still increasing when the concentration of glucose is 5 mM. (K_m is the substrate concentration at which the enzyme has reached half of its maximum rate of reaction, or 1.0 relative enzyme activity.)

11. d. The molar quantities of the different gene products need not be the same (because of different efficiencies of initiation of translation).

12. b. An inducible operon is turned off in the absence of the effector (inducer) molecule, and a repressible operon is turned on in the absence of the effector (co-repressor molecule). The effect of the inducer on operon activity is negative, although positive inducible operons have been described as well.

13. a. Mutation of the operator (O^-) in one chromosome would remove gene repression in that copy because the repressor protein cannot bind to the operator. In the second chromosome, *lacZ*, *lacY*, and *lacA* are mutated so they are not expressed. Also, the wild-type operator in that chromosome (O^+) cannot negatively regulate the wild-type gene copies in the other chromosome because the operator cannot act *in trans* (it only acts *in cis*).

14. c. This is the correct choice. In the first step of RACE, the synthesis of negative-strand cDNA depends on a polydT primer binding to the polyadenylation tail in mRNAs.

15. d. RACE requires reverse transcriptase to make DNA from RNA, whereas PCR requires DNA polymerase (to make DNA from DNA).

16. c. Northern blotting is a technique to detect RNA, whereas the products of RACE are cDNAs.

17. d. The distance between two genes (in the map unit of Morgan) is equal to the sum of the recombinant frequencies in the progeny:
$$0 \times \left(\frac{37}{100}\right) + 0 \times \left(\frac{46}{100}\right) + 1 \times \left(\frac{11}{100}\right) + 1 \times \left(\frac{7}{100}\right)$$
$= 0.18$ Morgan, or 18 centimorgan.

18. d. This choice is correct. There are three possible crossover events: one crossover between the first and second gene, one crossover between the second and third genes, and a double crossover. These events would give rise to a total of six different recombinant phenotypes (which, in the table, are all the phenotypes other than wild-type and crossveinless, echinus, scute). Single crossovers would separate the first or third genes from the other two, whereas the double crossover event would allow the gene that is in the middle to assort independently of the first and third genes. Because a double crossover event occurs much more rarely than a single crossover, the phenotypes that are much less frequent must be the ones where the middle gene phenotype occurs independently of the other two genes' phenotypes (cv-sc and ec), revealing which gene is in the middle: the ec gene.

19. a. The exchange event occurs during the prophase of the first meiotic division.

20. b. As stated in the passage, chiasmata are sites where chromosomes remain together after a crossover event. There is one chiasma in the WT image and there are five in the syp-1–depleted image.

21. d. All interferons have antiviral properties, including interferon-γ, although its primary action is to activate macrophages. Loss of interferon-γ is associated with decreased resistance to bacterial infection and tumors.

22. a. As stated in the article that reported this figure, "Analysis of 120 healthy individuals revealed a highly significant difference of female and male PBLs [cells] to produce IFN-α after TLR7 stimulation with R848 (Fig. 2A; $p < 0.0000001$, two-tailed Mann-Whitney U test). In contrast, IFN-α induction in the same females and males after TLR9 stimulation with CpG-ODN 2216 did not differ significantly (Fig. 2B), indicating that preferential IFN-α induction in female subjects is TLR7 dependent."

23. c. As stated by Meier et al., "plasma progesterone levels were significantly correlated to the percentage of IFN-α$^+$ pDCs following [HIV-1] stimulation." Levels of progesterone rise during the luteal phase of the menstrual cycle.

24. c. The likelihood of nonwhite women starting ART is statistically lower ($p < 0.05$) than that of white men.

25. b. IFN-α plays a central role in hepatitis C virus infection, which disproportionately affects men.

26. b. This is the correct choice. Staurosporine is an apoptosis stimuli that causes mitochondria to fragment.

27. c. These steps take place in the mitochondria in eukaryotes. However, aerobic bacteria carry out this process in the cytosol.

28. c. NADH (and FADH$_2$, not shown in the illustration) is a carrier of high-energy electrons.

29. d. The fundamental feature that distinguishes most forms of necrosis from apoptosis is the rapid loss of cellular membrane potentials.

30. b. Superoxide anion (O_2^-) is the precursor of most ROS.

31. a. Several groups have addressed the issue of causation using an mtDNA polymerase with eliminated proofreading activity and the polymerase activity preserved.

32. b. As stated in the passage, it has been speculated that tissues with the highest energy demand are also the most susceptible to mitochondrial mutations. Gastrointestinal tissue has relatively low energy requirements.

33. b. Actin filaments support the transport of cellular material but over much shorter distances than microtubules.

34. d. The top junction is the tight junction.

35. c. Rotavirus protein VP4 induces changes of the subapical actin network as the virus enters cells. An apical point of entry could be reasoned because the virus is gastrointestinal. Because HCV is a blood-borne virus, it enters through the basolateral domain.

36. c. Adding the soluble extracellular domain of a cell junction protein over time disrupts trans-epithelial resistance. However, expressing this domain inside cells would not be predicted to have an effect because this domain would have to be on the outside of the cell.

37. b. Antibodies targeting E2 and SR-BI and soluble heparin only strongly inhibit entry when added during the binding phase of infection; these factors all play a role in HCV host cell binding. Antibodies targeting CD81 block infection when added pre- or post-binding, indicating that these agents block post-binding HCV cell entry events.

38. c. Penetration decreases the risk for immuno-detection because no viral proteins remain exposed on the plasma membrane.

39. c. Incineration is a method to destroy prions and decontaminate materials.

40. b. Antibodies can selectively target misfolded proteins while sparing native, properly folded protein if, as stated in the passage, native protein has important functions in the cell.

41. d. Misfolding of prion proteins is associated with a change from soluble alpha-helical conformation to beta-sheet-rich aggregates.

42. c. The aerobic oxidation of glucose forms 30 to 32 ATP molecules.

43. d. Acute pancreatitis is caused by the inability of the pancreas to secrete zymogens to the intestine. As a result, zymogens are converted to their catalytic active form inside the pancreas, which attacks the pancreatic cells.

44. b. This reaction is endothermic, so $\Delta H > 0$. Also, two moles of gas has less entropy than three moles, so $\Delta S > 0$.

45. c. Flavoproteins that are fully reduced (two electrons accepted) generally have an absorption maximum near 360 nm, whereas they acquire another absorption maximum at about 450 nm when partially reduced (one electron).

46. b. 16-carbon palmitic acid goes through seven passes through the oxidative sequence, and the overall result is the conversion of the 16-carbon chain of palmitate to eight 2-carbon acetyl groups of acetyl-CoA molecules.

47. a. Progesterone has a ketone group (R_2CO), whereas testosterone has an alcohol group (OH).

48. c. As explained in organic chemistry, the thick line represents the trans conformation, whereas the dotted line represents the cis conformation.

49. d. Osmotic pressure can be calculated using the osmosis equation $\pi = i\,M\,R\,T$, where π is osmotic pressure, i is the Van 't Hoff factor, M is molarity, R is the gas constant (0.08206 L atm mol^{-1} K^{-1}), and T is temperature.

50. c. The TIM22 complex is located on the inner membrane of the mitochondria, not the cell surface.

51. a. The conversion of IPP to terpenoids begins with isomerization to DMAPP.

52. c. The graph shows the highest percentage of dMBP staining, which is an indicator of myelin degeneration, for tissues from individuals with VaD (vascular dementia).

53. a. Immunostaining is based on antibody recognition of an antigen. (In the case of this passage, the antigen is degraded myelin basic protein [dMBP].)

54. b. The force that it would take an ion such as Na$^+$ to go spontaneously through an ion channel is ΔG, represented by the equation $\Delta G = RT \ln (C \text{ inside}/C \text{ outside}) + Z F V_m$, where R is the gas constant, T is the temperature, $C\ inside/C\ outside$ is the ratio of the concentration of the ion inside and outside the cell, Z is the ion charge, F is the Faraday constant, and V_m is the difference in electrical potential. $\ln (C \text{ inside}/C \text{ outside})$ is -2.395.

55. a. The depolarization of cells caused by the opening of Na$^+$ channels causes K$^+$ channels to open, and the K$^+$ efflux repolarizes the membrane locally.

56. d. Neurons and endocrine cells respond to extracellular calcium, which is a second messenger, by triggering exocytosis.

57. c. The two types of bones have the same mineral and matrix components.

58. d. As stated in the footnoted article, the main function of the liver is to process the nutrients absorbed from the small intestine.

59. d. The Wnt/Wingless pathway is important for the differentiation of hair.

Part 2: Chemical and Physical Foundations of Biological Systems

1. a. As an approaching source moves closer during the period of a sound wave, the effective wavelength shortens, and the pitch (frequency) increases accordingly, since the velocity of the wave is unchanged. This is an example of the Doppler effect. The pitch of a receding sound source will be lowered per the Doppler effect, and the Venturi effect describes fluid velocity in a pitot tube or a constricted pipe.

2. a. According to Newton's second law ($\vec{F} = m\vec{a}$), the acceleration of the wagon is equal to the net force divided by the mass of the wagon ($\vec{a} = \frac{\vec{F}}{m}$). To determine the net force, the force of friction must be added to the horizontal component of the applied force. The force of friction is given in the question (100 N), so the horizontal component (in the x direction) of the applied force must be determined. Answer **b** would be obtained if *sin* was used rather than *cos*.

$$\vec{F}_{horizontal} = \vec{F}\cos(\theta) = (240\ N)\cos 50.0°$$

$$= 1.54 \times 10^2\ N$$

$$\vec{a} = \frac{\vec{F}}{m} = \frac{\vec{F}_{horizontal} + \vec{F}_{friction}}{m}$$

$$= \frac{1.54 \times 10^2\ N + (-100\ N)}{500\ kg}$$

$$= 0.108\ m/s^2$$

$$= 10.8\ cm/s^2$$

3. c. The half-chair conformation is more stable than the planar conformation, but it is the least-stable non-planar conformation for cyclical hexoses. The half-chair conformation is less stable than the boat conformation, the chair conformation is the most stable cyclic carbohydrate conformation, and the twist-boat conformation is more stable than both the boat and half-chair conformations, but it is less stable than the chair conformation.

4. c. This molecule is a benzene ring with two substituents, CH_3 and F, located on adjacent carbons on the benzene ring.

The benzene ring of the molecule contains four hydrogen atoms altogether, and each has a unique set of connections to carbon atoms, which means there are four unique hydrogens and four proton NMR signals contributed by the benzene ring. The methyl group contributes one additional unique hydrogen, giving a total of five unique hydrogens and therefore five proton NMR signals. There are four unique hydrogen atoms on the benzene ring and one unique hydrogen atom on the methyl group in this molecule, so there are five total proton NMR signals. The two substituents on benzene are different, giving four unique sets of connections on attached carbons. Additionally, each hydrogen atom on the benzene ring is bonded to a carbon that has a unique set of connections, so there are four unique hydrogen atoms and therefore four proton NMR signals produced by the 2-methylfluorobenzene ring. There is one additional proton NMR signal produced by the one unique kind of hydrogen on the methyl group. Finally, the molecule contains five unique hydrogens and therefore five proton NMR signals.

5. d. The calculation is shown below:

$$\text{molality} = \frac{\text{moles of solute}}{\text{kg of solvent}} = \frac{1.0 \text{ kg} \times \dfrac{1{,}000 \text{ g}}{1 \text{ kg}} \times \dfrac{\text{mol}}{342 \text{ g}}}{400 \text{ mL} \times \dfrac{0.791 \text{ g}}{1 \text{ mL}} \times \dfrac{1 \text{ kg}}{1{,}000 \text{ g}}}$$

$$= 9.2 \text{ mol} / \text{kg}$$

Choice **a** is the molarity, not the molality; **b** is the molarity value with the molality units; and **d** is the molality value with the molarity units.

6. c. Hydrophobic moieties are most likely to interact with the hydrophobic interior of CDs. The internal cavity of a CD is hydrophobic, so positively charged molecules are not the most likely moieties to interact with the inside of a CD cylinder, because the internal cavity of a CD is hydrophobic, negatively charged molecules are less likely to interact with this portion, and although amphipathic molecules have hydrophobic portions, purely hydrophobic moieties are most likely with the hydrophobic interiors of CDs.

7. d. The weak base neutralizes the HCl that the reaction generates, and the reaction is an $S_N 2$ reaction. A weak base is needed to neutralize the HCl generated by the reaction. Adding a weak acid will not accomplish this. Also, the reaction is an $S_N 2$ reaction, not an $S_N 1$ reaction. Answer **b** is an $S_N 2$ reaction, not an $S_N 1$ reaction, and a weak acid, not a weak base, must be present to neutralize the HCl that will be generated in this reaction.

8. c. The CDs replace the tosyl groups on the nanoparticles, as shown in Figure 1. This occurs because tosylate is a good leaving group. Sulfonic acids generally make for excellent leaving groups because their conjugate bases are quite stable. Tosyl groups essentially act as placeholders, preventing reactivity and also serving as leaving groups for substitutions. No oxygens are contributed directly by the tosyl group. The sulfur from tosyl does not contribute to the functionalized final product, and tosyl groups are commonly used as protecting groups; here the tosyl groups would not encourage PEG hydrolysis.

9. c. This structure can be seen in Figure 2. There is a C = O stretching peak at 1710 cm^{-1}. There is also a key band at 1,535 cm^{-1} that is caused by the –NH bending vibration in the amide linkage between the silane and the PEG, which is not present in any of the other species in the answer choices. Additionally, the 1,280-cm^{-1} peak corresponds to the Si–C stretching vibration, which should not be present in any of the other species. Less obvious but still useful are the 1,595-cm^{-1} characteristic benzene ring vibration and the 817-cm^{-1} benzene ring bending vibration. Therefore, there are a number of ways to distinguish this spectrum from the other answers. The distinct peak at 1,710 cm^{-1} indicates the presence of a carbonyl group. As PEG diol contains no carbonyl groups, choice **a** can be ruled out. Additionally, a number of key peaks are missing, including the peaks at 1,595 cm^{-1} for characteristic benzene ring vibration and at 817 cm^{-1} for benzene ring bending vibration. The Si–C and –NH peaks at 1,280 and 1,535 cm^{-1} are also absent. Finally, the distinct peak at 1,710 cm^{-1} indicates the presence of a carbonyl group, which would not be present in the final β-CD-PEG-MNP product. Additionally, the glycosidic bond in β-CD-PEG-MNP causes a number of peaks; specifically, peaks at 943.9 cm^{-1} (α-pyranyl vibration) and 1151/1077/1029 cm^{-1} (C-O-C glycosidic bridge stretching vibration) are not present in this spectrum that would be present in the spectrum for β-CD-PEG-MNP.

10. d. This is the structure of L-kynurenine. The name of the enzyme, indoleamine 2,3-dioxygenase, describes exactly where the reaction occurs on L-tryptophan, with oxygen insertion occurring accordingly. The passage explains that the formyl group is subsequently removed from *N*-formylkynurenine, which results in this molecule, L-kynurenine. Choice **a** is the structure of melatonin, **b** of L-tryptophan, the reactant in the IDO1 reaction, and **c** of dopamine.

11. b. The technique allows *His*-tagged proteins with an affinity for the metal ion to be retained in the nickel column. Protein separation is not based on size, anion exchange resins do use positively charged groups, the binding principle here is based on affinity, not charged interactions, and cation exchange resins use negatively charged groups to attract positively charged proteins.

12. a. The best buffer selection is the one whose pK_a is within 1 pH unit of the desired pH. The only buffer in the table with a pK_a within 1 pH unit of the desired pH, 6.5, is potassium phosphate, which has 7.20 as its most useful pK_a. The pK_a of potassium acetate, Tris, and TEA are all not within 1 pH unit of the desired pH of 6.5.

13. b. The Lineweaver-Burk plot is a double reciprocal plot that graphs $1/v$ as a function of $1/[\text{substrate}]$. The Eadie-Hofstee diagram represents enzyme kinetics by plotting reaction rate as a function of the ratio between rate and substrate concentration, the Hanes-Woolf plot represents enzyme kinetics by plotting $[\text{substrate}]/v$ against $[\text{substrate}]$, and the Hill plot, based on the Hill equation, quantifies the cooperativity of ligand binding to a macromolecule by describing the fraction of macromolecule saturated by ligand as a function of the ligand concentration.

14. a. Figure 1B shows that $V_{\max}$ remains constant and K_m increases, so it is competitive inhibition. $V_{\max}$ and K_m decrease in uncompetitive inhibition, $V_{\max}$ decreases and K_m stays the same in noncompetitive inhibition, and there is no evidence of irreversible covalent adduct formation here.

15. a. Schwann cells are the main glial cells of the peripheral nervous system. Myelinating Schwann cells wrap around axons to form the myelin sheath. Presynaptic cells are the cells at the synapse that release neurotransmitters to stimulate the postsynaptic cells, postsynaptic cells are cells that take up neurotransmitters at the synapse, and Langerhans cells are dendritic cells in the skin that capture and process microbial antigens in skin infections in order to become antigen-presenting cells.

16. d. Sphingolipids contain a sphingosine backbone that is O-linked to a head group, which is usually charged. This perfectly describes galactocerebroside, which has a galactose head group. Sterol lipids include cholesterol and are all derived from the same fused four-ring core structure, glycerolipids include triglycerides and mono-, di-, and tri-substituted glycerols, and fatty acids are carboxylic acids with long aliphatic chains that can be saturated or unsaturated.

17. b. The large ligand on the hydroxyl at carbon 1 is easily most stable in the equatorial formation. Moving around the galactose ring would also place the sulfated galactocerebroside in the equatorial position. Having both larger cyclical hexose ligands in the equatorial position is the most stable configuration. If the sulfated hydroxyl group at carbon 3 is axial, the large ligand on carbon 1 is also axial. This is extremely unstable, the equatorial configuration for the sulfated hydroxyl and the large group at carbon 1 is far more stable than the axial configuration for the groups. Therefore, both are not equally stable, and there is no benzene ring in the structure. The ring is a cyclohexose.

18. b. The strong separation of charge by the myelin sheath greatly limits ion leakage and effectively decreases the number of ions that must be pumped back after each action potential. The myelin sheath does not cause any kind of diffusion of sodium and potassium ions across the axon, there is no relationship between the increased propagation speed and any work done by the axon, and choice **d** is effectively a statement of Bernoulli's principle as it applies to fluids, but it is irrelevant to this system because the myelin sheath does not decrease the pressure of the axon as a means of increasing impulse speed.

19. c. A dielectric material is an electrical insulator that can be polarized by an applied electric field. A semiconductor is a solid substance with a conductivity between that of an insulator and a conductor. The passage states that myelin is an insulator, so this cannot be correct. A cathode is an electrode, and the role of myelin as an insulator indicates that

this is not the correct answer. And a refrigerant causes cooling, which is in no way the function of myelin.

20. c. Statements I and III are correct, but statement II is incorrect because the work done by a force in a conservative system is independent of the path taken.

21. b. A path can be constructed from the starting point to the finishing point that features a horizontal line across and a vertical line down. The horizontal displacement is perpendicular to the downward gravitational force, so no work is done here, but in the vertical displacement, the work done is equal to mgh. According to the work kinetic energy theorem, the net work done causes an increase in velocity, and since the skier began at rest, it can be stated that $mgh = \frac{1}{2}m(v_f)^2$. The mass value cancels out on both sides of this equation, and the equation can be rearranged as $v_f = \sqrt{2gh} =$

$$\sqrt{2 \times (9.8\tfrac{m}{s^2}) \times (15.0\ m)} = \sqrt{294}$$

$= 17.1$ m/s.

22. d. For a conservative system, the change in potential energy is equal to the negative amount of work done. If we imagine a horizontal and vertical path from the starting point to the ending point of the skier's journey, we can assume that no work is done horizontally because the path is perpendicular to the gravitational force, but for the vertical path, the work done is equal to mgh. That means that the change in potential energy is equal to $-(55.0\ kg) \times (9.8\tfrac{m}{s^2}) \times (15.0\ m) = -8{,}085\ J = -8.09$ kJ.

23. c. Kinetic energy is equal to $\frac{1}{2}m(v)^2$, which in this conservative system is equal to mgh. Since m and g are constant, the highest kinetic energy will be observed when there is the greatest difference in starting and ending heights. This occurs at height 0 m. The skier will either be motionless or just picking up speed at the top of the first hill. Halfway down the first hill h is equal to 45 m, and the skier reaches the maximal speed at height zero between the hills. The skier will lose kinetic energy as she ascends the next hill.

24. a. This question is essentially asking which of these amino acids is basic (although binding can also occur to aromatic amino acids), and of the four, arginine is the only one that fits the bill. Histidine and lysine residues are also basic residues and likely candidates to receive an electron from the dye. Glutamic acid is acidic, so it would not receive a proton from the dye, cysteine is not basic and would not receive a proton from the dye molecule, and glutamine is not basic, so the dye would not readily donate a proton to cysteine.

25. c. Binding of dye to the hydrophobic pockets occurs via van der Waals forces, while amine binding to negatively charged dye functional groups occurs via ionic interactions. Hydrogen bonds are not essential here. The structure of the dye reinforces this idea, with only a limited number of possible H-bond donors or acceptors.

26. d. The standard curve line equation, determined using the known protein solutions, can be used to calculate the concentration of the protein of interest because the Bradford assay functions the same way on all proteins, regardless of identity. For general characterization of a protein, determining the molecular weight is important, and size-exclusion chromatography is the way to determine this value. However, the molecular weight will not be useful for calculating the protein concentration. The mechanism by which the dye binds the protein does not matter because the A_{595} is measured after binding is complete. The spectrum of the red form of the dye is not needed for any kind of correction of the measured A_{595} value.

27. c. The Bradford assay is nonspecific in its interaction with proteins. Therefore, the Bradford assay will detect all proteins, not just the one protein of interest. The molar absorptivity is specific to the one protein of interest. In order to use the Beer-Lambert law, an accurate A and c must be determined for the protein of interest, which means that the protein must be extremely pure. Otherwise, the calculated molar absorptivity will not be accurate. The presence of cofactors should not influence molar absorptivity determination using the Beer-Lambert law, the protein will lose its quaternary structure when bound to the dye, so the polymeric form is not essential here, and the Bradford assay is not reliant on tryptophan residues; its source of absorbance is not intrinsic to the protein but rather results from the bound dye.

28. c. SDS is regularly used for cell lysis, a critical step in the protein purification procedure. SDS detergent is not commonly used in cell growth media; while it is true that SDS is used for protein separation in SDS-PAGE, SDS-PAGE is not part of a standard purification procedure because it denatures the protein. Once a protein sample undergoes the SDS-PAGE procedure, it is not used for purposes like finding concentration via the Bradford assay—and SDS is not needed to stabilize most chromatographic resins.

29. a. The red and green forms of the dye have a positive charge, and SDS is an anionic detergent. SDS associates strongly with the red/green form of the dye, causing the dye equilibrium to shift. More of the blue form of the dye is produced, causing an increase in absorbance at 595 nm, independently of protein presence. This is the mode of Bradford assay disruption at high SDS concentrations. Based on Le Châtelier's principle, the absorbance should increase, not decrease; based on Figure 1, anionic SDS is unlikely to associate strongly with the negatively charged blue form of the dye, and anionic SDS is unlikely to associate strongly with the negatively charged blue form of the dye.

30. b. SDS can bind to the protein via van der Waals forces and ionic interactions, inhibiting protein binding sites for the dye reagent and causing underestimation of the protein concentration because the dye is not able to bind protein to its full extent. The detected absorbance is therefore too low, and the concentration is underestimated. This is the mode of Bradford assay disruption at low SDS concentrations. SDS binding to the protein inhibits protein binding sites for the dye reagent and causes underestimation, not overestimation, of the protein concentration. It also will block protein-dye interactions— it is not likely to enhance interactions due to the bulkiness of all molecules involved.

31. c. When it comes to absorbance spectra, dyes of each color will have maximum absorbance wavelengths that correspond with its opposite color on the color wheel. In other words, absorption in the visible region gives the complementary color. According to this principle, the red form of the dye will have a maximum wavelength in the green range (450 to 560 nm), whereas the green form of the dye will have a maximum wavelength in the red range (640 to 700 nm). Even without an electromagnetic spectrum at hand, the order of the three colored dyes' wavelengths of maximum absorbance can be determined based on theory alone. 250 nm is UV light, not visible light, and the reverse of choice **d** is true.

32. c. $\Delta A = 2\alpha A \Delta T = 2\left(\frac{18.9 \times 10^{-6}}{°C}\right)\left(\pi\left(\frac{10.0}{2}\right)^2 cm^2\right)$ $(50.0°C) = 0.148\ cm^2$. The hole will change in size when the brass is heated and answer **d** would be obtained if one used 10.0 cm as the radius rather than the diameter.

33. b. Buoyancy describes the ability of something to float in a fluid and is not relevant here. Water progresses up the xylem tubes via transpirational pull, and it is the surface tension of water that forms the meniscus, pulling water up the xylem. Cohesion describes the ability of molecules or small particles to hold together. Interactions between water molecules create the surface tension that makes capillary action possible. And adhesion describes the ability of molecules or small particles to stick to a surface or object. Here, it is just as important as cohesion, because adhesion promotes interaction between the water molecules and the wall of the xylem.

34. b. $r = \frac{mv}{qB} \rightarrow B = \frac{mv}{qr}$

$= \frac{(1.67 \times 10^{-27} \text{ kg}) \times (7.50 \times 10^7 \text{ m/s})}{(1.60 \times 10^{-19} \text{ C}) \times (1.00 \text{ m})} = 0.783 \text{ T}$

35. d. The K_{sp} value is a constant and will stay the same, and $PbCl_2$ solubility will decrease because the addition of more chloride to the solution will shift the equilibrium to the left, increasing the amount of solid $PbCl_2$, per the common-ion effect. The K_{sp} value will not be affected by ion concentrations.

36. b. α particles are positively charged, which is consistent with the observations in this experiment. The atomic nucleus is positively charged, so neutrons would not be repelled by the nuclei, β particles are negatively charged, which is inconsistent with repulsion by the nuclei, and γ particles have a neutral charge, so they would not be repelled by the positively charged nucleus.

37. a. The first three ionization energies become increasingly larger, but the fourth ionization energy is extremely large because the full electron shell of Al^{3+} makes it very unlikely that Al^{4+} will form. Ionization energies measure electron removal, not electron addition. Electron addition is described by electron affinity. No electron excitation is involved in ionization energy trends and, in many cases, energy and mass are inversely proportional, but this is irrelevant to the ionization energy trends. Additionally, no significant mass changes are taking place.

38. c. $q_{sucrose} = q_{water} + q_{calorimeter}$

$= mc\Delta T_{water} + mc\Delta T_{calorimeter}$

$= (600 \text{ g})(4.18 \text{ J/g} \cdot °C)(10.0°C) + (250 \text{ g})$
$(20.0 \text{ J/g} \cdot °C)(10.0°C)$

$= 75.1 \text{ kJ}$

$n = \frac{q_{sucrose}}{\Delta H_{sucrose}} = \frac{75.1 \text{ kJ}}{5.65 \times 10^3 \text{ kJ}} = 0.0133 \text{ mol sucrose}$

$0.133 \text{ mol sucrose} \times \frac{342.30 \text{ g}}{\text{mol}} = 4.55 \text{ g sucrose}$

Choice **a** would be obtained if only the q_{water} value was used to determine n, **b** if only the $q_{calorimeter}$ value was used to determine n, and **d** if the specific heat capacities were swapped in the equation.

39. b. Residual activity is lowest in the presence of constant DCCD when the Na^+ concentration is lowest, and residual activity increases as Na^+ activity increases. The activity of the ATPase is highest when no DCCD is present, confirming its role as an inhibitor, but Na^+ protects against the inhibition by DCCD. Based on the data, Na^+ is not an inhibitor of the ATPase; in fact, the data show that the ion combats inhibition of the ATPase by Na^+. DCCD inhibits ATPase, but Na+ protects against its inhibition based on the data. Therefore, the two molecules do not work cooperatively to inhibit the enzyme. Finally, comparing the DCCD-free control to any of the trials that include DCCD shows that DCCD is an inhibitor, and increasing the concentration of Na^+ protects against this inhibition.

40. a. Faraday's laws of electricity are two-fold, and this is an accurate statement of the first of the two laws. The quantities are directly proportional, not inversely proportional, and while capacitance is the ability of a system to store electric charge, this is not relevant to Faraday's laws.

41. c. Statement II is correct because liquids have more entropy (disorder) than solids, and statement III is correct because the melting of ice is an endothermic process. Statement I is false because ice melting at 55°C is spontaneous.

42. c. The ideal gas law assumes molecules are point masses with no volume and with no intermolecular attractions. The van der Waals equation corrects for both of these factors. Phase changes would not be an issue in a system that only involves gases, and chemical bonding is not a factor that the van der Waals equation covers, neither of these factors in choice **b** is covered by the van der Waals equation, and the ideal gas law already accounts for molecular masses, as well as pressure in general.

43. d. Gel filtration chromatography, also called size-exclusion chromatography, separates proteins based on size. Because calmodulin I and hemoglobin are so similar in size, the UV-Vis detector at the bottom of the column would likely detect overlapping peaks that would be difficult to separate without optimization of the technique. Paper chromatography separates molecules on paper based on polarity. The passage describes a size-based method, so this is not an appropriate choice. Additionally, SDS-PAGE denatures proteins. The passage describes a method where the proteins recovered after size-based separation were collected for further purification and structural analysis, so SDS-PAGE could not have been used. Finally, distillation separates liquids based on boiling points. This technique is not relevant to this protocol.

44. a. The original protein solution can be poured into a dialysis tube, which would then be sealed and placed into a large container of the new buffer. This would be allowed to sit for a few hours, allowing the buffers to exchange. Repeating this process several times allows for nearly complete buffer replacement. Affinity chromatography is irrelevant here; HPLC allows for molecule separation but not buffer exchange; and extractions separate solutes based on distribution between two immiscible solvents—this is not a method for buffer exchange.

45. b. At a pH above the pI, proteins carry a net negative charge. The pH, 5.0, is higher than the pI of calmodulin I. Calmodulin I will carry a net negative charge and will therefore bind to the positively charged anion exchange resin. At a pH above the pI, proteins carry a net negative charge. The buffer pH (5.0) is lower than the pI of hemoglobin. Hemoglobin will carry a net positive charge and will therefore *not* bind to the positively charged anion exchange resin. Only calmodulin I will bind to the resin. Hemoglobin will not, and calmodulin I will bind to the resin, even though hemoglobin will not.

46. d. The Soret peak is caused by π-π^* transitions in the porphyrin ring, which is the heme bound to hemoglobin. The passage indicates that heme is bound to hemoglobin because after the heme cofactor was added, hemoglobin successfully bound oxygen. The secondary structure of the protein does not cause this particular UV-Vis peak, and tryptophan absorbance occurs at 280 nm, not the 412-nm Soret peak described in the passage.

47. d. The calculation below shows how this answer is obtained using Hess's law of heat summation.

$$C_2H_6\,g \rightarrow C_2H_2\,g + 2HC_2H_6(g) \rightarrow C_2H_2(g) + 2H_2(g)$$
$$\Delta H = +94.5 \text{ kJ}$$

$$2CO_2(g) + 3H_2O(g) \rightarrow C_2H_6(g) + \tfrac{7}{2}O_2(g)$$
$$\Delta H = +283 \text{ kJ}$$

$$2H_2(g) + O_2(g) \rightarrow 2H_2O(g)$$
$$\Delta H = -2 \times 71.2 \text{ kJ} = -142.4 \text{ kJ}$$

$$2CO_2(g) + H_2O(g) \rightarrow 1C_2H_2(g) + \tfrac{5}{2}O_2(g)$$
$$\Delta H = +235 \text{ kJ}$$
$$\times 2$$

$$4CO_2(g) + 2H_2O(g) \rightarrow 2C_2H_2(g) + 5O_2(g)$$
$$\Delta H = +470 \text{ kJ}$$

Choice **a** would be obtained by adding together the three ΔH values as they are currently, without any manipulation, **b** if one failed to multiply the overall equation by 2 after the other equations have been added together, and **c** if one failed to multiply the third equation by 2.

48. a. The limiting reactant is CO_2, based on the calculations below, and 2.0 g of CO_2 produces 0.59 g C_2H_2.

$$4CO_2(g) + 2H_2O(g) \rightarrow 2C_2H_2(g) + 5O_2(g)$$

$$2.0\,g\,CO_2 \times \tfrac{mol}{44\,g} \times \tfrac{2\,mol\,C_2H_2}{4\,mol\,CO_2} \times \tfrac{26\,g}{mol} = 0.59\,g\,C_2H_2$$

$$2.0\,g\,H_2O \times \tfrac{mol}{18\,g} \times \tfrac{2\,mol\,C_2H_2}{2\,mol\,H_2O} \times \tfrac{26\,g}{mol} = 2.9\,g\,C_2H_2$$

$2.0\,g\,H_2O \times mol\ 18\,g \times 2\,mol\,C_2H_{22}\,mol\,H_2O \times 26\,g\,mol = 2.9\,g\,C_2H$. Choice **b** would be obtained if a 1:1 mole ratio was assumed between CO_2 and C_2H_2, when in fact the correct mole ratio is 4:2, **c** if the mole ratio between CO_2 and C_2H_2 is flipped from 4:2 to 2:4, and **d** is the theoretical yield from 2.0 $g\,H_2O$; however, CO_2 is the limiting reactant, so the C_2H_2 yield should be calculated from the 2.0 $g\,CO_2$ reactant.

49. c. The number of gas molecules increases over the course of the reaction, increasing the disorder of the system and therefore resulting in a positive ΔS. ΔS does not rely on the ratio of reactants involved in the reaction, and because the number of gas molecules increases over the course of the reaction, ΔS will be positive, not negative.

50. d. The calculation is shown below, in which the chemical equation is used to find the number of moles produced, and then that number of moles is used in the ideal gas equation to solve for the volume.

$$4CO_2(g) + 2H_2O(g) \rightarrow 2C_2H_2(g) + 5O_2(g)$$

$$5.00\,g\,CO_2 \times \tfrac{1\,mol\,CO_2}{44\,g\,CO_2} \times \tfrac{5\,mol\,O_2}{4\,mol\,CO_2} = 0.142\,mol\,O_2$$

$$V = \frac{nRT}{P} = \frac{(0.142\,mol) \times (0.08206^{L\cdot atm/mol\cdot K}) \times 273\,K}{1.00\,atm} = 3.18\text{ L}$$

Choice **a** would be obtained if 32 K was used instead of 273 K, **b** if the CO_2:C_2H_2 mole ratio was used instead of the CO_2:O_2 mole ratio, and **c** if a 1:1 mole ratio was used.

51. d. There are two ligands on the central carbon and no lone pairs. There are no lone pairs on the central carbon in CO_2 that would cause the bent shape, there are not four ligands on the central carbon, and the T-shaped geometry occurs when there are three ligands and two or three lone pairs. Since there are only two ligands and no lone pairs on CO_2, this cannot be the correct shape.

52. b. Unlike resistance, resistivity is a material constant for a particular material and is independent of sample dimensions. State functions refer to thermodynamic functions that depend only on the current state of the system, Figure 1 shows that resistivity is temperature dependent, but resistance is also temperature dependent, and resistance (R) and resistivity (ρ) are related by the equation $= \frac{\rho L}{A}$.

53. b. XRD is based on constructive interference of monochromatic X-rays and a crystalline sample. When the X-rays are directed at a sample, the diffracted rays are collected, with the angle between the incident and diffracted rays being a crucial feature of all diffraction. X-ray diffraction (XRD) does not provide information about the reactivity of the film, spectroscopic techniques are more apt to serve this purpose, but XRD does not detect excited electrons, and though Ni-O bond lengths and bond angles are indeed structural features of NiO films, it is not the purpose of XRD.

54. d. In semiconductors, as temperature increases, more electrons receive kinetic energy and are excited from the valence band into the conduction band. Increased thermal energy therefore increases current and decreases resistivity (per Ohm's Law). As temperature increases in a semiconductor, resistivity decreases, which is what is seen in Figure 1. The Figure 2 graph is also typical of semiconductors. Conductors tend to increase their resistivity with an increase in temperature—this is the opposite of what is seen in Figure 1—the data here are unrelated to the magnetic properties of NiO, and insulators are essentially semiconductors with a huge band gap, which means they would require a tremendous temperature change for excitation into the conduction band. The resistivity should therefore remain high and constant until this high temperature change is achieved. Figure 1 shows that resistivity starts to decrease immediately at 30°C, which is not characteristic of an insulator.

55. a. Based on the units used on the plot, the activation energy is equal to the slope of each line multiplied by the Boltzmann constant (in eV), the y-intercept does not provide a valid means to determine the activation energy, the x-intercept does not provide a valid means to determine the activation energy, and this sum does not provide a valid means to determine the activation energy.

56. b. A purine is a heterocyclic aromatic compound consisting of an imidazole ring fused to a pyrimidine ring. Based on Figure 1, this perfectly describes adenosine. Porphyrins are heterocyclic conjugated ring systems, a pyrimidine is an aromatic heterocycle with a 1,3-diazine (pyrimidine) core— it only has one ring, rather than the two fused rings a purine has—and a flavin is a naturally occurring pigment that has a tricyclic aromatic molecular structure.

57. c. An exergonic reaction proceeds with a net release of free energy, so ΔG is negative for an exergonic reaction. It is true that ATP hydrolysis is exothermic, but this cannot be stated based solely on the ΔG value. ΔG is a measure of the change in Gibbs free energy. The word *exothermic* is based on ΔH. Additionally, $\Delta G^{\circ\prime}$ describes the change in Gibbs free energy, not the change in enthalpy, and an endergonic reaction has a positive $\Delta G^{\circ\prime}$, and the ATP hydrolysis reaction has a negative $\Delta G^{\circ\prime}$.

58. a. $\Delta G_{\text{erythrocytes}} = \Delta G^{\circ\prime} + RT\ln K = \Delta G^{\circ\prime}$

$+ RT\ln\dfrac{[\text{ADP}][\text{P}_i]}{[\text{ATP}]} = -30.5^{\text{kJ/mol}} +$

$(0.008314^{\text{kJ/mol·}K})(310\ K)\ln$

$\dfrac{(0.25 \times 10^{-3}\text{M})(1.65 \times 10^{-3}\text{M})}{2.24 \times 10^{-3}\text{M}} = -30.5^{\text{kJ/mol}} +$

$(2.58^{\text{kJ/mol}})(-8.6) = -30.5^{\text{kJ/mol}} + (-22^{\text{kJ/mol}})$

$= -52^{\text{kJ/mol}}$

Choice **b** would be obtained if the concentrations for ATP and ADP were swapped in the K calculation, **c** if the temperature was left in °C rather than Kelvin, and **d** if the inverse K was used.

59. c. There is actually greater solvation of these molecules relative to ATP, making it significantly easier for ATP to lose one of its phosphate groups. The repulsion of the like charges on ATP is a major reason why breaking the phosphoanhydride bond is so exergonic, resonance stabilizes ADP more than ATP, which contributes to making ADP a more stable molecule than ATP, and the higher disorder and lower free energy in ADP relative to ATP thermodynamically explains the observed $\Delta G^{\circ\prime}$.

Part 3: Psychological, Social, and Biological Foundations of Behavior

1. b. The amygdala controls anger and rage. The occipital pole controls vision, the cerebellum controls physical coordination, and the fornix carries signals through parts of the brain.

2. d. Venting to other people about the parking problem is an example of an emotion-focused strategy. In emotion-focused coping, the person attempts to remove the anxiety brought about by the stressful situation. The man attempts to reduce his anxiety by venting to friends. Problem-focused coping involves taking control of the situation that is causing stress—approaching the neighbor is an example of problem-focused coping—while speaking with the apartment complex manager is a direct way of taking control of the situation and thus also an example of problem-focused coping. Writing a letter to the apartment association would be the execution of a plan to take control of the stressful situation and is another example of problem-focused coping.

3. c. The parietal lobe receives and processes sensory information from the body. The frontal lobe controls problem solving and decision making, the occipital lobe is the visual processing center, and the temporal lobe regulates memory.

4. a. The olfactory pathways carry the sense of smell from the nose to the brain. The optic nerve carries transduced light from the eyes to the brain, nerves at the base of the tongue carry the sensation of taste to the brain, and sounds travel through many parts of the ear before reaching the nerves that carry them to the brain.

5. a. Damage to the frontal lobe would most affect higher-level cognition. Damage to the occipital lobe would most affect visual processing, damage to the parietal lobe would most affect sensory information from the body, and damage to the temporal lobe would most affect memory.

6. a. Cognitive dissonance occurs when new experiences conflict with expectations, causing initial confusion and dissatisfaction. The passage states that the cognitive dissonance was not primarily a problem with the students in the class. Cognitive dissonance would not make the supervisors happy, and there is no indication of complaints from other student teachers.

7. a. This study was focused on a single subject and therefore was a case study. This study had a sample size of $n = 1$ and thus was not a traditional experimental or a split-half design, and as data collection was via videotape and interview, there were no items to equate.

8. b. The supervisors expected the graduate student to conform to their traditional way of teaching. There was no indication of peer pressure in this study; role playing is practice, whereas this was an actual classroom; and social loafing would require the student teacher to be working in a group, when in fact she was working alone (except with the researcher, who would not be a part of the group in a social loafing situation).

9. c. The graduate student's decision to persevere despite her supervisors' cognitive dissonance is an indication of high self-efficacy. Self-fulfilling prophecy was not a factor in this study, stereotypes were not a factor in this study, and stigma was not a factor in this study.

10. d. The reference group would be all the other teachers of the biology course, past and present. The concept of class identity was not a factor in this study; the self-identity would belong to the graduate student, not the supervisors; and the power group in this case would be the supervisor.

11. c. Parallel processing would allow the brain to determine the color of the dress and differs among people, so one person's brain might see blue and black and another's would see white and gold. Somatosensation deals mostly with other areas of the body, including the organs, skin, and joints; the color of the dress has already been determined before it reaches the optic nerve; and auditory processing is associated with the ear and hearing.

12. a. The hormones in the endocrine system are responsible for the fight or flight phenomenon. The lymphatic system creates immune cells, the integumentary system is responsible for exocrine glands, like skin, hair, and nails, and the cardiovascular system circulates blood around the body via the heart, arteries, and veins, delivering oxygen and nutrients to organs and cells, and carrying their waste products away.

13. b. These beliefs are likely to begin turning around at age 5 to 7 due to brain development. These beliefs are still strong during the age 4 to 6 range, have already started to turn around before the age 8 to 9 range, and start to change much younger than the age 10 to 11 range.

14. c. Eastern cultures tend to value their elderly because of the wisdom they provide, whereas Western cultures tend to value youth because of their appearance and health. Western cultures also offer financial incentives to the elderly, such as Medicare and senior discounts, aging is socially constructed in both the East and the West, and Eastern cultures tend to take the view that nursing homes show neglect of their elderly family members.

15. d. This is a valid argument to the statement given in the stem. The statements in **a** and **c** are misinformed, and while **b** is a commonly heard objection, it is not related to the question.

16. b. Facebook involves two-way (or more) interactions between people and in some cases groups; thus, it is the largest contributor to the social construction of reality of all the answer choices given. Television generally communicates in one direction, and although it adds to the social construction of reality in some instances, it is not the best answer. Satellite radio may contribute to the social construction of reality, but compared to Facebook, it is a much smaller contributor. And a computer server is the technology behind computer networking, but it does not directly provide a social environment.

17. a. Colleague A is observing Colleague B for many years and is using the information to guide his future attitude toward him. Vygotskian theory focuses primarily on the development of children, which does not apply to this situation, social conflict theory has wealth and economics as its basis, and rational choice theory suggests that people always make logical decisions that provide them with the greatest benefit and are in their highest self-interest.

18. c. The agent of socialization in this case is the workplace. There is no deviance present in this relationship, collective behavior includes large groups of people, not just two people, and this is about individual interaction, not the larger social norms.

19. a. Colleague A's emotions toward Colleague B adapt as he provides support to Colleague B after he loses his job. Universal emotions relates to facial expressions showing emotions, the adaptation of emotions in this passage occurs during adulthood, and the brain has completely developed by age 35.

20. d. The limbic system houses the emotions. The cerebellum deals with physical balance, the cerebral cortex is the covering of the brain and deals with memory and perceptual awareness, and the brain stem deals with systems that keep humans alive.

21. c. Piaget developed the larger theory of equilibration that included accommodation. James and Lange studied emotions, Maslow developed the hierarchy of needs, and Vygotsky viewed learning as socially, not individually, constructed.

22. b. Assimilation means the brain changes the new information to fit existing knowledge. Accommodation is when the brain changes its structure to fit the new knowledge, equilibration includes both assimilation and accommodation, and stage progression is not a psychology term.

23. c. The difference in students' scores from pre- to post-test is the dependent variable in the study. The students who received the conceptual change instruction were the experimental group, **b** is the independent variable, and the teacher who did NOT provide the instruction was in charge of the learning of the control group.

24. a. When learners go through the process of challenging their misconceptions, they often experience cognitive dissonance, which is described in the stem of the question. While there is some negative feedback involved, the BEST theory to fit the model is cognitive dissonance. In the behaviorist model, teaching goes from teacher to student based on the *tabula rasa* idea—challenging misconceptions is not part of behaviorist instruction—and the biopsychosocial approach is within the paradigm of illness and medicine and not part of the conceptual change model.

25. d. The educational system is the agent of socialization MOST responsible for resistance to change, because most instruction goes from teacher to student and the conceptual change model includes the student to a much greater extent. The student is expecting to be told the science concepts, not have them challenged. Although science concepts may be talked about in the home, the school is most responsible for a student's resistance to change; the media may have some effect on the student's resistance to change, but the school's influence is much greater; and peers are likely to have little effect on a student's resistance to change.

26. d. Dissatisfaction is most likely to invoke attitude change because of the emotions involved in having misconceptions challenged. Intelligibility is unlikely to invoke any attitude change. Depending on the concept (e.g., evolution), there may be a significant attitude change, but this is likely to be the case with only a few concepts, so *dissatisfaction* is a better answer. And while fruitfulness may invoke happy feelings, the attitude change will be far less than with dissatisfaction.

27. c. This is an example of bottom-up processing using perceptional inputs. Choices **a**, **b**, and **d** are examples of top-down processing.

28. a. Breast development in boys occurs in response to rising estradiol levels. The opposite of **b** is true, menarche is the first onset of menstruation in girls, and myelinization occurs in the brains of boys and girls.

29. b. The basic idea of a fundamental attribution error is to think someone's intentions are malicious when they are not. The example in choice **a** is the opposite of a fundamental attribution error, **c** has more to do with self-concept than a fundamental attribution error, and **d** is a self-fulfilling prophecy, not a component of a fundamental attribution error.

30. c. The Internet is not a social institution. Parts of the Internet are used in mass media, which is often considered a social institution, but the Internet itself is not. Marriage is part of the family and, thus, a type of social institution; education includes schools, which are social institutions; and government is a social institution.

31. a. Autophagy impairment as described in the passage would be slowed in neuron cells. Autophagy impairment as described is slowed, not speeded up; cell destruction would not occur abruptly, as this is a long-term process; and if cell destruction stopped altogether, the patient would become terminal.

32. c. Autophagy (protein misfolding) would increase the personality disorder behaviors. Mania symptoms would increase when autophagy is impaired, Parkinson's disease symptoms would worsen, and drug abuse is often associated with autophagy impairment.

33. a. The control group did NOT receive the therapy. The treatment group DID receive the therapy, choice **c** is a description of a dependent variable, not the control group, and the researchers performing the study were not a group in the study.

34. c. Social reproduction relates to systems that keep generations of a family within the same social status. Intersectionality relates to intersections of systems of oppression, class consciousness relates to the beliefs of an individual about his or her class status, and intergenerational mobility relates to social status change within a family.

35. a. Privileged status is based on inheritance of property; oppressed status is based on reproducing new workers. Oppressed status is based on reproducing new workers, not the maintenance of the privileged women, privileged women are also oppressed, and the status of privileged women is not based on human reproduction.

36. b. Both are higher than in the privileged class.

37. a. Oppressed women often do not have access to quality health care because of where they live and a lack of transportation. The illness experience is a description of the stages or sequence of being ill, medicalization is the process through which a specific illness becomes an illness in the medical community, and the sick role can change a person's social status during his or her illness.

38. d. One group is being discriminated against by another group. In this passage, no aggression is evident, in-group and out-group deal with the individual, not the group, and prejudice has to do with bias.

39. d. The best practice would be to keep all variables the same and repeat the experiment with a new set of subjects. The proper procedure would be to continue to investigate the same problem, it would not be good experimental practice to reuse the same groups when repeating the experiment, and when repeating the experiment, both groups should be the same size.

40. a. The looking-glass self theory states that a person's identity is an outgrowth of his or her interactions with others and perceptions. Role taking is when a person takes on the role of another person to interpret a situation, imitation is when a person's identity comes from imitation of others, and reference group is not an identity formation theory.

41. b. Differential association theory does not explain why individuals become criminals. Strain theory focuses on why they become criminals, collective behavior focuses on the group, not the individual, and labeling theory is associated with the development of a sense of self in all people, not just criminals.

42. b. Interpersonal attribution has to do with interactions between two or more persons. External attribution has to do with the surrounding events; although common sense is a component of attributional theory, there is no such thing as common sense attribution; and correspondent inference has to do with how individuals make sense of situations—there is no psychological concept called correspondent inference attribution.

43. a. Because the methodology led to an improvement in intergroup functioning, it can be hypothesized that the use in trying to reduce prejudice may be fruitful. Because the methods had a positive effect on the participants, it is unlikely that they would reduce self-efficacy; the passage states that the third-person perspective improved the outcome, so it is unlikely to affect the inter-actions in a negative way; and cognition is likely to be increased when these methods are used.

44. d. The first-person and third-person perspectives were the independent variables in the research study. The control group is the group that received no treatment, the experimental variable is the group that received the treatment, and the dependent variables are looked at to determine the outcome of the research study.

45. a. The name of the experimental group in sociological terms is the primary group. The secondary group is most likely the group the primary group visualized interacting with, the out-group refers to a group of excluded people, which does not apply to any group in this study, and a triad consists of three people and does not apply to this study.

46. c. The learning in the experimental group is occurring through modeling and observation. Classical conditioning does not occur in this study, there are no rewards or punishments in this study, and no reinforcement schedules are used in this study.

47. b. The correct term in this case is *consensus*, because all of the participants performed the same. Consistency refers to a single individual's consistency of performance or thought, distinctiveness would have to do with a single person being distinct from the others, and expectation does not apply to this experiment.

48. a. *Labeling* is a synonym for *stigma* in this passage. Stereotyping typically comes from outside one's cultural group; ethnocentrism is judging a cultural group outside one's own; and self-fulfilling prophecy is the opposite of what is occurring here.

49. b. The woman is having symptoms of bipolar disorder that she cannot control. She is ignoring her illness, which means she is avoiding health care, is avoiding experiencing a sick role, and is avoiding letting others know she is sick and thus is not relying on others for help.

50. d. Mood swings are common in individuals with bipolar disorder. Forgetfulness is a sign of dementia-type diseases such as Alzheimer's and Parkinson's, and although some individuals with advanced bipolar disorder might experience psychosis, including hearing voices, as well as delusions, this patient is having mild symptoms.

51. a. It is a social norm in some cultural groups to ignore symptoms of illness because of the stigma attached. Deindividuation relates primarily to large groups such as crowds, social facilitation is the phenomenon where performance is altered due to the presence of another person or other people, and the bystander effect is when a group of people witness a person in need of help but do not attempt to help.

52. d. Environmental factors, including events that are few and far between, such as earthquakes and floods, are unlikely to induce change around the stigma of disease. Spread of disease is a biotic factor and is likely to cause social change around the illness experience, birth and death rates from particular diseases are likely to influence cultural views of disease, and ideology about diseases can cause social change about the stigma that surrounds them.

53. b. There was a control group for each race. If the researchers wanted to increase the number of patients used in the study, they would add more patients to the original two subgroups; the various symptoms could be compared using one subgroup each; and if the results were not as expected, the researchers would most likely run a follow-up study to investigate the findings.

54. c. The typical neuron has four major parts. It may look like there are two, three, or five parts in some of the images, but in the typical neuron, there are four.

55. d. *Soma* is another name for the cell body. Axons conduct electrical impulses away from the neuron's cell body or soma, dendrites conduct electrical impulses toward the neuron's cell body or soma, and the function of a process is to be a conduit through which signals flow to or away from the cell body.

56. a. The man's symptoms indicate a possible diagnosis of bipolar disorder, which is most likely caused by disruptions in neurotransmitters. The brain stem is not the location of the biological processes that cause mental illness, mental illness is not caused by disruptions in the soma, and disruptions in the processes do not cause mental illness.

57. a. Absolute threshold decreases with age. Although auditory pathways relate to hearing, choice **b** is not why the child hears something the adult does not hear, feature detection is related to vision, and choice **d** is not an example of signal detectors.

58. b. Reinforcement schedules are a part of operant conditioning. Variable ratio reinforcement is not a part of classical conditioning, choice **c** is an example of behavioral learning, not cognitive learning, and **d** is not an example of modeling.

59. a. Source monitoring errors occur when a recollected experience is incorrectly determined to be the source of the error. Neuroplasticity is the brain's ability to change based on experience, trace decay error is the fading of short-term memories over time, and interference occurs when long-term memories are interfered with by new information.

Part 4: Critical Analysis and Reasoning Skills

1. a. The opening sentences set up the idea that a large body of Haydn's work has been neglected and that what *is* played is "perfunctorily performed."

2. c. While the term *picturesque* usually describes something visual, like a painting or a landscape, Saint-Saëns has described how the sounds of the musical composition mimic sounds in nature, almost as if you could imagine the natural scene as you listen.

3. b. One of the specific innovations Saint-Saëns mentioned in the passage was Haydn's use of the clarinet, which had previously only played a "humble role" in the orchestra.

4. b. Saint-Saëns emphasizes that once Haydn began creating music for a larger audience in London, his musical genius took "magnificent flights," implying that a change in his circumstances is what allowed his genius to flourish.

5. c. Saint-Saëns spends a lot of time describing the images of the music of Haydn. This statement most closely aligns with his views of Haydn's *Seasons*, so it is likely he would agree with this statement.

6. a. The letter portrays a composer whose imagination and ideas proliferate despite his declining health and physical ability to do his work. This seems to support Saint-Saëns' view of Haydn as prolific, with a wealth of imagination.

7. d. In the opening paragraph, Madison mentions the lack of intellectual rigor in Goldman's writing, but elsewhere in the passage he does not focus on this flaw as an overarching problem for the movement.

8. d. Madison examines Goldman's belief that what is natural to a government is unnatural to the individual and that government fundamentally goes against human nature.

9. d. In the final paragraph, where Madison discusses Goldman's legacy as the "daughter of the dream," he mentions that "modern conditions" favor centralization but is vague as to the nature of those conditions. However, it is logical to conclude that reality (whatever the conditions of reality may be) has gotten in the way of the idealism of anarchism.

10. d. This society sounds closest to Goldman's definition of anarchy, which values "social wealth" or the "common good."

11. d. Goldman's philosophy is most critical of government and its negative effects on the lives of individuals. Her definition of anarchism emphasizes the "free grouping" of individuals to produce "social wealth." While Goldman's definition does advocate for a social group, it also advocates for the interests of the individual.

12. a. Goldman discusses protesting social conditions through the "assertion of economic power." Both Goldman and the protesters share a concern for economic disparity.

13. c. This answer is closest to the meaning of the passage. Sinclair describes the process of pork making as "some horrible crime committed in a dungeon, all unseen and unheeded, buried out of sight and of memory," and then begins to philosophize about the hog's poor existence.

14. c. When faced with the hog's death, over and over again, Sinclair (along with his readers) is forced to consider the hog's death more closely to give it meaning, which is the main purpose of the final paragraph.

15. d. The mention of a "god of hogs" is a wish that the hog could have some alleviation of its suffering and that its life and death had meaning.

16. c. This choice most closely addresses what Sinclair is doing in the final paragraph, which is to anthropomorphize the hogs.

17. c. The sentence sets up an equation between the treatment of the hogs and the working conditions of the man. To bring the discussion back to the reality of the farm strengthens Sinclair's overall purpose in exposing the conditions of the industry.

18. d. The passage focuses on the misery of the hogs and likens the process to some "horrible crime committed in a dungeon," which sounds similar to the "horror film" Jonathan Safran Foer describes here.

19. d. Rizal discusses a number of issues that led to the fall of the Spanish empire, so this is the most likely choice.

20. b. A pathology is an illness, so the metaphor suggests a dysfunction in the way Spain was led. Rizal cites Rome, another empire that enjoyed a great rise and a sharp decline, as well as Spain's history as teachable lessons in "how not to rule a country."

21. c. Rizal speaks in metaphor when he discusses both the priest and the soldier; they are symbols of war and religion. In this paragraph, Rizal moves between the literal and the metaphorical quickly and even mixes metaphors, but the overall intent of his paragraph is that neither religion nor war helped the advance of the Spanish culture—in fact, they hurt the empire.

22. a. In framing the piece of literature as the Spanish empire's "proudest hour," Rizal acknowledges that something good arose from this empire in decline but also portrays it as a singular event. Mentioning the fact that Cervantes was a soldier who lost one hand makes it seem like the war-waging empire failed to aid this writer but that he created the masterpiece in spite of his injury. The fact that the literature is an exaggeration of the country's defects supports Rizal's view that the empire suffered from many flaws.

23. c. In context, Rizal emphasizes a country that mourns the loss of what it once had.

24. d. The first flaw of the Spanish empire mentioned in the passage is corruption.

25. c. Osler emphasizes three main qualities—steadfastness, a desire for knowledge, and an open heart—in addition to other qualities, like humility and honesty.

26. d. In context, Osler does not simply compare the lunatic with the student but groups them together with the lover and the poet. The lunatic clings to an idea, whereas the student is "aflame with desire." The word "fervent" seems the closest in meaning to Osler's point.

27. c. Osler's emphasis is on how "every truth has to struggle to acceptance." Harvey's idea of blood circulation is an obvious truth now but had to be very carefully introduced to physicians.

28. a. Osler emphasizes that the thirst for knowledge, the quest for the truth, is more important for the student than being concerned with the end result—the "fervent longing" is the "be-all and the end-all."

29. a. Osler makes the point in the second paragraph that all truth has to "struggle to acceptance" as a warning to the student against what he calls "mind-blindness" but also to describe the process of sharing truth with the rest of the world (as in the case of Harvey).

30. a. The author's discussion seems to portray a student as one who loves the process of learning as much as the end results.

31. d. The term "corporate" commonly refers to business corporations but in this case simply means "group."

32. a. The final paragraph emphasizes that people can act without being fully aware of their motives.

33. b. The authors set up a comparison between a simple example of a man with a stone hammer who is natural and artificial at the same time to the more complex example of the extension of a group.

34. c. In Aristotle's view of society, it is an instinctual aspect of the human that "man is made for life in society."

35. a. Jung's ideas, which offer an explanation of unconscious motives, strengthen the idea that a group may be moved by unconscious motives.

36. b. While the symphony is made up of players, the harmony is a group of notes that exists beyond human consciousness.

37. b. The vast veil is a separation along racial lines, which speaks to the crux of W.E.B. Du Bois's main topic of discussion.

38. a. The metaphor is about looking beyond the artificial racial barriers set up in society. The sky was bluest when Du Bois succeeded and excelled at things despite facing racism.

39. b. The "problem," as Du Bois outlines in his discussion, disproportionately affects the black community, but this image indicates that it is a problem for all society.

40. d. The "color line" is similar to the "veil" Du Bois described earlier and pinpoints the issues of the relationship between blacks and whites. While he frames the issue as being a problem, the "problem" discussed in the quote is very similar.

41. a. Du Bois spends time discussing the invisible barrier that separates blacks from whites and would probably not insist that such a separation is logically impossible.

42. c. Engels describes the crowding of the city, saying that the people who live there have been "forced to sacrifice the best qualities of their human nature" and goes into some detail about how the city instills a sense of indifference within them.

43. b. Turmoil means commotion or disturbance, and this is what the author most closely means in context.

44. d. Even when Engels speaks of the city's view of the Thames with a certain amount of awe, it is described as impressive but also imposing. He does not highlight many beneficial aspects of the city.

45. c. In creating great things, the things of civilization, which is the advanced state of human society, Engels argues that human beings have had to sacrifice their best qualities and that as many as a "hundred powers" within human beings have been suppressed.

46. d. Engels mentions walking through slums, which may reflect a society that is characterized by "narrow self-seeking." The homeless shelter is a public good that has little to do with selfishness and may be one sight that would have countered the author's views.

47. a. The monkey's fight for dominance in its troop is similar to the "social war" Engels describes and the "strong treading the weaker underfoot."

48. a. S.G.W. Benjamin spends a good amount of time discussing a particular work of Eakins's, but the discussion begins with an attempt to characterize a new movement in art, moves on to include work by a couple of other painters, and concludes with a description of the characteristics of the movement.

49. b. This is the issue Benjamin pinpoints. After analyzing the image of an operation and mentioning other artists of the "horrible," he declares he will leave the question of whether or not it is right to show such a subject up to the public.

50. c. The purpose of the essay is to discuss and define a new movement in American art. Therefore, Benjamin must focus on it. Benjamin also, in fact, does mention artists of other cultures (i.e., Ribeira and Regnault).

51. c. Benjamin critiques things like perspective and lighting, which suggests the "new movement" is inclined toward realism, valuing how accurately the artist represents her subject.

52. c. The differences between the two compositions are the lighting and the establishment of antiseptic practices. If Eakins was a realist painter, then he may have been capturing the reality of the lighting of darker-lit figures.

53. a. Benjamin spends most of his time discussing the Eakins painting, and his critique focuses on how accurately the painter captured his subject in terms of perspective, lighting, and color.

ADDITIONAL ONLINE PRACTICE

Using the codes below, you'll be able to log in and access additional online practice materials!

Your free online practice access code is:
FVE1M38SYX722WT767DS

Follow these simple steps to redeem your code:

- Go to **www.learningexpresshub.com/affiliate** and have your access code handy.

If you're a new user:

- Click the **New user? Register here** button and complete the registration form to create your account and access your products.
- Be sure to enter your unique access code only once. If you have multiple access codes, you can enter them all—just use a comma to separate each code.
- The next time you visit, simply click the **Returning user? Sign in** button and enter your username and password.
- Do not re-enter previously redeemed access codes. Any products you previously accessed are saved in the **My Account** section on the site. Entering a previously redeemed access code will result in an error message.

If you're a returning user:

- Click the **Returning user? Sign in** button, enter your username and password, and click **Sign In**.
- You will automatically be brought to the **My Account** page to access your products.
- Do not re-enter previously redeemed access codes. Any products you previously accessed are saved in the **My Account** section on the site. Entering a previously redeemed access code will result in an error message.

If you're a returning user with a new access code:

- Click the **Returning user? Sign in** button, enter your username, password, and new access code, and click **Sign In**.
- If you have multiple access codes, you can enter them all—just use a comma to separate each code.
- Do not re-enter previously redeemed access codes. Any products you previously accessed are saved in the **My Account** section on the site. Entering a previously redeemed access code will result in an error message.

If you have any questions, please contact LearningExpress Customer Support at LXHub@LearningExpressHub.com. All inquiries will be responded to within a 24-hour period during our normal business hours: 9:00 A.M.–5:00 P.M. Eastern Time. Thank you!

NOTES